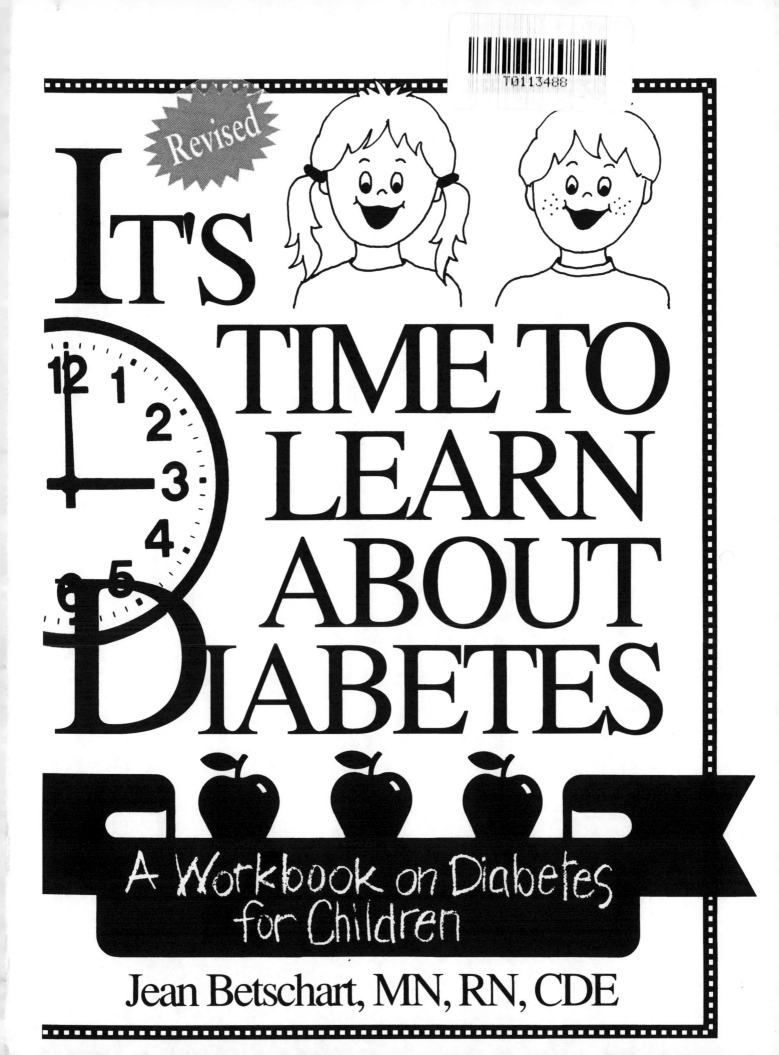

Revised

It's Time to Learn About Diabetes

A Workbook on Diabetes for Children

Jean Betschart, MN, RN, CDE

It's Time to Learn About Diabetes
Revised

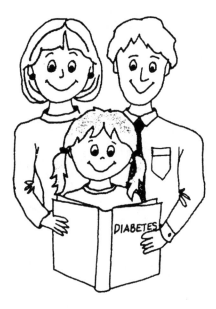

A Workbook
on Diabetes for Children

by Jean Betschart, MN, RN, CDE

Illustrations by Nancy Songer, RN, MSN, CPNP

The development of this work
was wholly supported by a grant from the
Diabetes Research and Education Foundation,
Bridgewater, New Jersey.

JOHN WILEY & SONS, INC.

Copyright © 1995 by Jean Betschart. All rights reserved
Published by John Wiley & Sons, Inc.
Published simultaneously in Canada
Previously published by Chronimed Publishing

To order books or for customer service please, call 1(800)-CALL-WILEY (225-5945).

The information contained in this book is not intended to serve as a replacement for professional
medical advice. Any use of the information in this book is at the reader's discretion. The author
and the publisher specifically disclaim any and all liability arising directly or indirectly from the
use or application of any information contained in this book. A health care professional should
be consulted regarding your specific situation.

ISBN: 978-0-471-34743-9

10   9

Acknowledgments

I greatly appreciate the support and encouragement of my colleagues in the Department of Endocrinology of Children's Hospital of Pittsburgh. I extend a special note of gratitude to Linda Siminerio, RN, MS, CDE, and Terri Yeager, RN, MSN, CRNP, CDE, for their interest in this project and especially to Nancy Songer, RN, MSN, CPNP, for her creative ideas and wonderful illustrations.

In addition, I want to thank the children who piloted the workbook and their families. They gave me "real" information on what a workbook should include!

I also am totally grateful for the loving support of my husband and family. Their tolerance of my endeavors has made it possible for me to find the time to complete the work.

Reviewers:

Dorothy Becker, MBBCH, FCD
Diane Betschart, teacher
James Betschart, DMD, PhD
Barbara Bodnar, RN, BSN, CDE
Theresa Byrd, RN, CDE
Pat Carroll, MD
CHP Patient-Parent Education Committee
Louisa Cohen, teacher
Patricia Cooper, teacher and parent
Lynn Crowe
Emma D'Antonio, RN, PhD
Dathleen Dwyer, RD, PhD
Nancy Johncola, RN, CDE
Tom Lantz, teacher and parent
Margretta Lockard, teacher
Melinda Maryniuk, RD, CDE
JoAnne Moore, RN, BSN, CDE
Anita Nucci, RD, CDE
Noreen Papathoradeau, MSW
Sandra Puczynski, RN, MS, CDE
Max Salas, MD
Linda Siminerio, RN, MS, CDE
Linda Steranchak
Terri Yeager, RN, MSN, CRNP, CDE

Table of Contents

Unit V: Doing Well During Special Times

Unit VI: On My Own

To the Teacher . . .

As an educator, nurse, dietitian or related professional, you have an instrumental role in shaping the lives of children with diabetes. This workbook is intended to enhance your role by serving to supplement classroom learning.

This is a level I book, intended for use by the newly diagnosed child with insulin dependent diabetes mellitus. It is targeted for children ages 8 to 10 years, or second through fourth grade who are performing at grade level without learning disabilities or developmental delay. The content will serve to reinforce classroom learning and is not intended to replace classroom experiences.

The workbook is progressive in that each chapter builds on previous knowledge. Optimal learning will take place if the chapters are completed consecutively.

Throughout this workbook, blood sugar levels are expressed in milligrams per deciliter. If you live in Canada, Great Britain, or elsewhere and measure blood sugar in millimols per deciliter, you will find the approximate converted figures for each example on page 104.

You, as an educator, should use discretion regarding the use of this workbook in terms of the length and intensity of assignments. Units or chapters might be assigned as homework between education sessions. It is unlikely that most children would be able to complete the workbook during the initial hospitalization.

Your student will most likely learn best if you take time to either work through the exercises or review them with the child. As teachers, we never fail to learn from our students' responses.

To the Parent . . .

Your task is a difficult one when it comes to creating a physically, mentally and emotionally healthy environment for your child. Sometimes compromises must be made with a sacrifice in one area to complement a need in another.

This workbook is intended to help to promote independence in your child. Knowledge of diabetes management is the first step in achieving independence. However, it is most important to keep in mind that children develop at very different rates. Therefore, what one child is able to accomplish at a given age, another child quite appropriately will not be able to do.

Encouraging your child to participate in his own self-care should not affect diabetes control. Supervision, involvement, continued interest and encouragement from parents is very important at all ages. Your child should **not** be expected to independently take care of his diabetes. Parental involvement has been shown to positively affect diabetes control.

If you are able to help your child work through this workbook or discuss chapters after your child does them, his or her learning and awareness of your interest will be that much greater.

Important Phone Numbers and Information

Doctor _____

Diabetes Educator _____

Dietitian_____

Pharmacy _____

Emergency_____

Child's Insulin Brand and Type _____

Size of Syringes_____

Meter Type_____

Strips _____

To the Student . . .

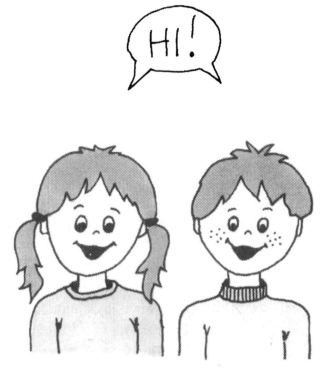

My name is Cindy and this is my friend Mike. We have diabetes. We're going to be your helpers as you do this workbook. We like knowing about diabetes so we can take care of ourselves and feel good! We know you're going to learn a lot. We sure did!

Your friends,

Cindy   Mike

Cindy and Mike

A Letter to my Friend . . .

Date _____

Dear _____,

You may be wondering why I came to the hospital and what is happening to me while I'm here. The doctors told me I have diabetes. The nurses wrote this letter for me to send to you so you can learn a little about diabetes. While I'm in the hospital, I'm learning how to take care of my diabetes, and I'd like to tell you about it.

Before I came to the hospital, I wasn't feeling well. Kids who have diabetes sometimes lose weight, feel tired and thirsty, and may have to go to the bathroom a lot.

Diabetes is NOT a disease like a cold or flu. No one can catch diabetes from me. What happened was that my body stopped making insulin. (Insulin helps my body use food for energy.) Now I will need to get my insulin with a syringe. Insulin makes the tired, thirsty feeling go away. It may sound terrible to you to have to take insulin every day, but if it will keep me healthy, it's worth it!

If I have too much insulin, exercise too much, or do not eat enough, my blood sugar level might get too low. That means there is not enough sugar in my blood. I may feel tired, grouchy, sweaty, shaky, dizzy, or confused. If that happens, I need to eat or drink something sweet, like orange juice, soda pop, or sugar tablets. I usually feel better in about ten minutes.

Another way I need to take care of my diabetes is by eating the right amounts of the right kinds of foods at the right times. I will eat healthy foods.

After I get home from the hospital, I can tell you more about what it was like, if you want to know. My diabetes won't keep me from doing anything. You can call or write to me at the hospital. See you soon!

Your Friend,

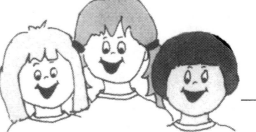

Name _____ Date _____

Chapter 1.

Diabetes: How Did I Get It?

Your body is made up of many parts. Each
part works with the others to keep you
healthy. Sometimes one part of your body
may not work as well as it should. When
this happens, you might not feel well.

**See if you know
what your body
parts do. I didn't!**

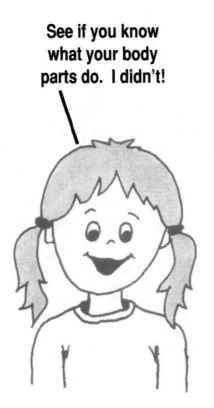

One part of your body, called your pancreas, has many jobs. One job the pancreas has is to make insulin.

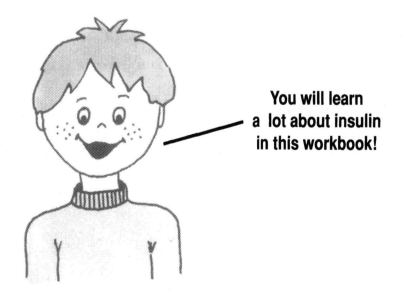

You will learn a lot about insulin in this workbook!

Look at the picture of some of the body parts inside you

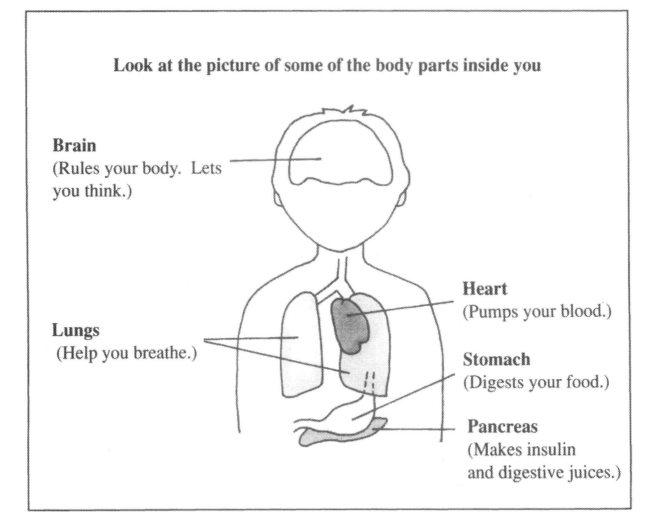

Brain
(Rules your body. Lets you think.)

Lungs
(Help you breathe.)

Heart
(Pumps your blood.)

Stomach
(Digests your food.)

Pancreas
(Makes insulin and digestive juices.)

Answer these questions:

    1. What body part lets you think?_____

    2. What body part digests your food? _____

    3. What body part makes insulin and juice to digest food? _____

    4. What body part helps you breathe? _____

    5. What body part pumps your blood? _____

**Draw the heart, lungs, stomach, brain, and pancreas
in the body outline below.
Write the names of each part and draw a line to it.**

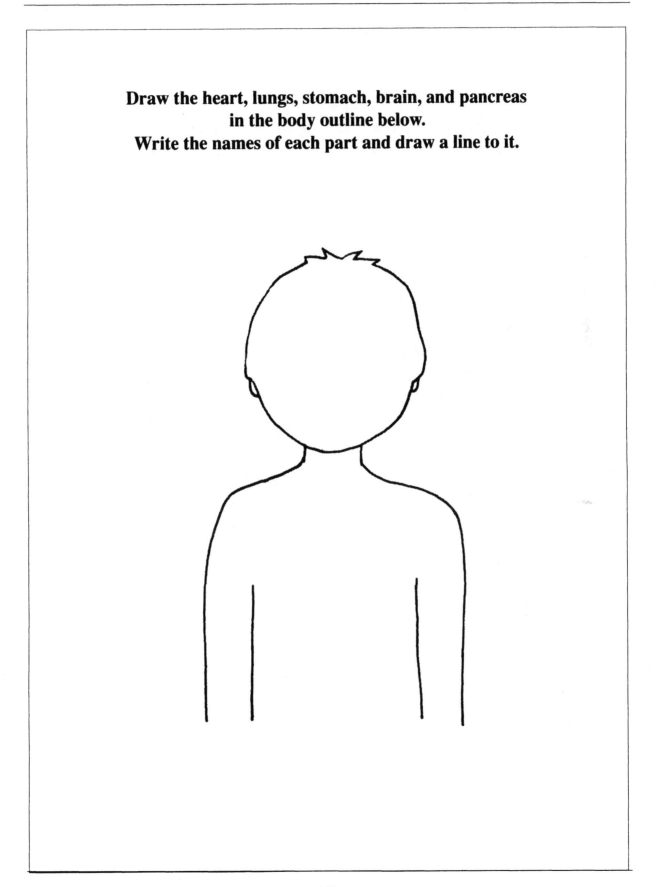

When your pancreas stops making insulin, you have diabetes.

What is the name of the illness that happens when your
pancreas stops making insulin? _____

You didn't do anything to cause your
diabetes. Diabetes is not caused by
eating or drinking too much sugar.
Sometimes a cold or flu can bring on
diabetes in some people who may be
going to get it, but you couldn't have
stopped diabetes from happening.

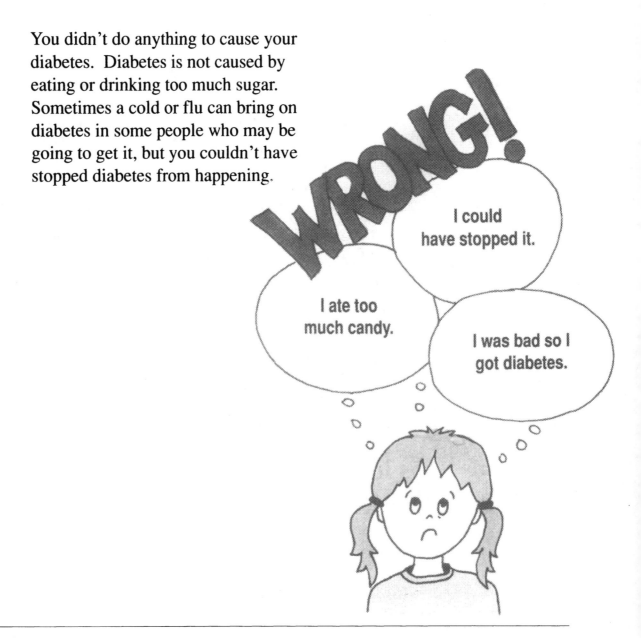

Circle the correct answer.

1. When you get diabetes, which body part has stopped making insulin?

   Lung   Heart   Pancreas   Stomach

2. Could you have kept yourself from getting diabetes?

   Yes   No

3. What can sometimes bring on diabetes in people who may be going to get it?

   Eating sugar   Drinking sugar   A cold or flu

Diabetes just happens.

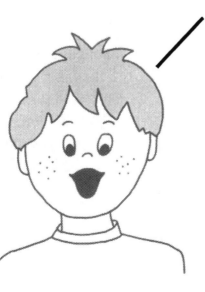

Name _____   Date _____

Diabetes: What does it mean?

Even when you have diabetes, most of your pancreas works
just fine. Only one small part of your pancreas stops making
insulin.

Insulin helps your body use food to give you energy. You need
energy to do all the things you do every day, like go to school and
play.

If your pancreas doesn't make
insulin, the only way to have
enough is to take it by using a
syringe.

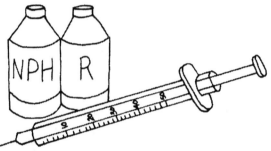

People who have diabetes must do special things, like take insulin,
to take good care of themselves so they will stay healthy.

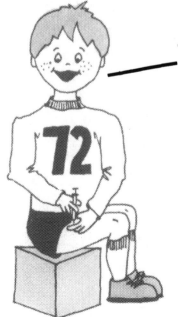

**Taking insulin really is OK!
Sometimes you might not
feel a thing when you take
your insulin, but other
times you might feel
a little pinch.**

You will need to eat well balanced meals and snacks on time. Most foods that don't have too much sugar or too much fat are OK to eat. Having foods with sugar in them can be worked into your plan.

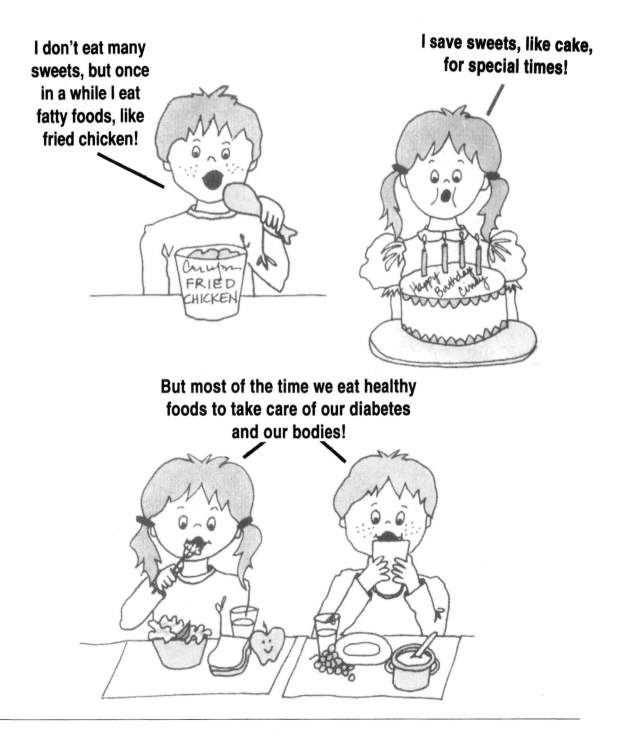

People with diabetes need to check their blood for sugar and their urine (pee) for ketones. We'll tell you more about ketones a little later.

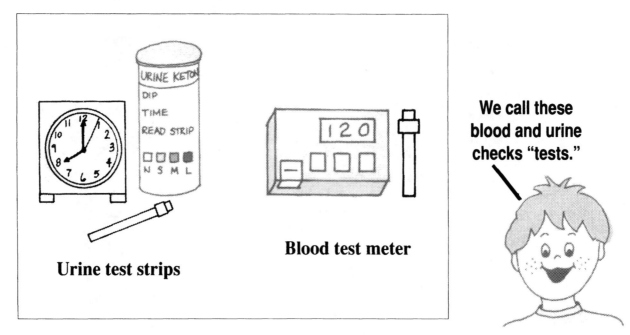

Urine test strips

Blood test meter

We call these blood and urine checks "tests."

It is important for you to learn how to do the test exactly right and to write down the numbers you get.

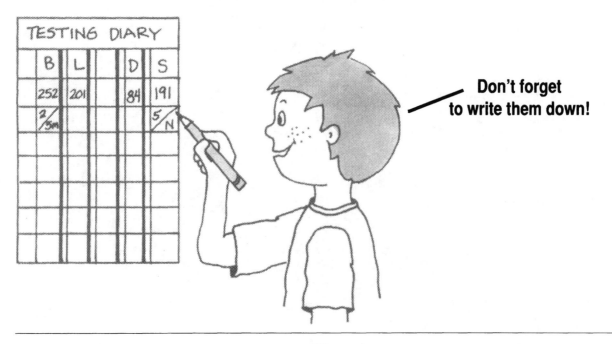

Don't forget to write them down!

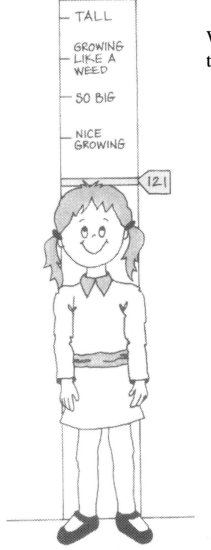

When children with diabetes take care of themselves, they feel healthy and grow just fine.

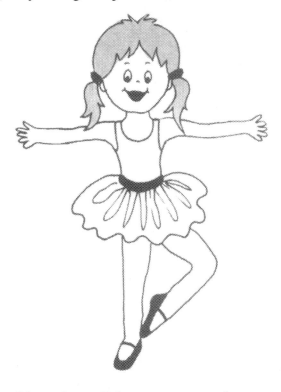

If you have diabetes, you can play
in all sports and activities!
Exercise is good for you!

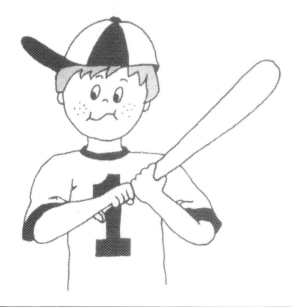

Circle 5 things that children with diabetes should do to take good care of themselves.

Skip meals   Take insulin

Test blood   Eat on time

Eat fatty foods   Test urine

Write down your blood and urine sugar numbers

In this puzzle, find these words:

INSULIN	PANCREAS	SUGAR	DIABETES
URINE	TEST	SYRINGE	HEALTHY
STOMACH	BODY	FAT	SNACKS
KETONE	EXERCISE		

U	D	T	W	N	V	X	S	O	Q	P	T	E	S	T
S	I	C	N	P	F	Q	L	S	A	P	E	E	W	Y
T	A	O	P	A	Z	X	C	N	B	G	M	K	H	G
O	B	Y	S	U	G	A	R	G	N	Q	S	P	O	I
M	E	O	N	B	G	F	T	I	A	S	D	A	S	C
A	T	N	D	Z	A	P	R	O	W	I	E	N	K	T
C	E	L	J	Y	M	Y	C	X	Z	A	S	C	E	G
H	S	X	L	P	S	O	E	S	S	V	Q	R	T	I
Q	U	I	E	G	I	N	S	U	L	I	N	E	O	H
A	S	R	I	R	C	X	V	B	N	M	N	A	N	Z
M	N	O	I	V	C	S	N	A	C	K	S	S	E	W
L	K	F	H	N	S	I	O	I	E	R	T	W	E	F
D	M	A	Y	X	E	J	S	K	P	L	T	Q	R	E
S	Y	T	B	O	S	L	H	E	A	L	T	H	Y	M
K	L	O	Z	Q	S	D	S	F	G	H	I	W	X	A

Name _____ Date _____

Chapter 2.

What Happens When You Get Diabetes?

Insulin works on your body cells. One job of your pancreas is to make insulin.

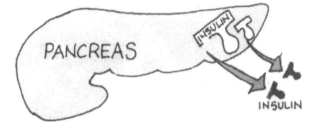

Did you know that your whole body is made up of cells?

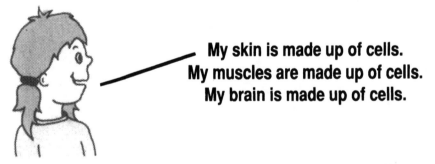

**My skin is made up of cells.
My muscles are made up of cells.
My brain is made up of cells.**

Cells are so small we can't see them with our eyes. Cells might look like this when you look through a microscope.

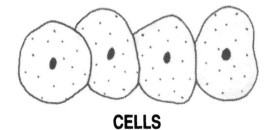

CELLS

Cells are alive because our bodies are alive! But they need to have sugar in order to live. Cells don't eat pizza, apples, or cheese. They eat sugar made from all the food you eat! Insulin lets sugar get inside the cells. Then you have energy to run, play, think, and do everything you do!

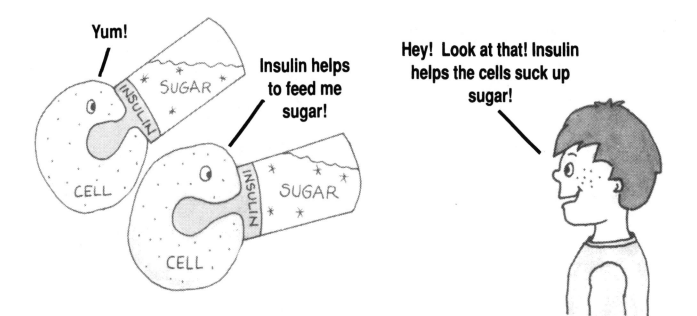

Each cell can eat when insulin helps sugar from the food you eat get inside. When cells are able to eat, they are happy.

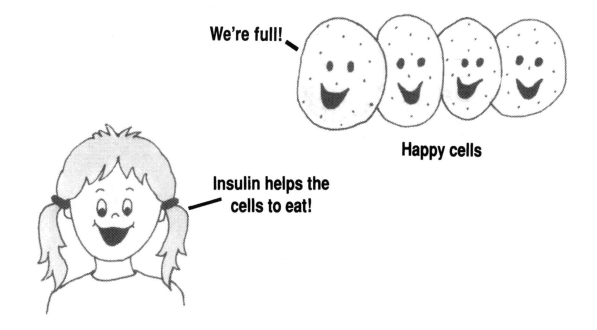

Fill in the missing letters for these words.

1. This body part makes insulin. __ __ N __ R __ A __

2. Your body is made up of these. __ __ L L __

3. Not made by your pancreas when you have diabetes. __ __ S U __ I __

4. Cells need to eat __ U G __ __ to live.

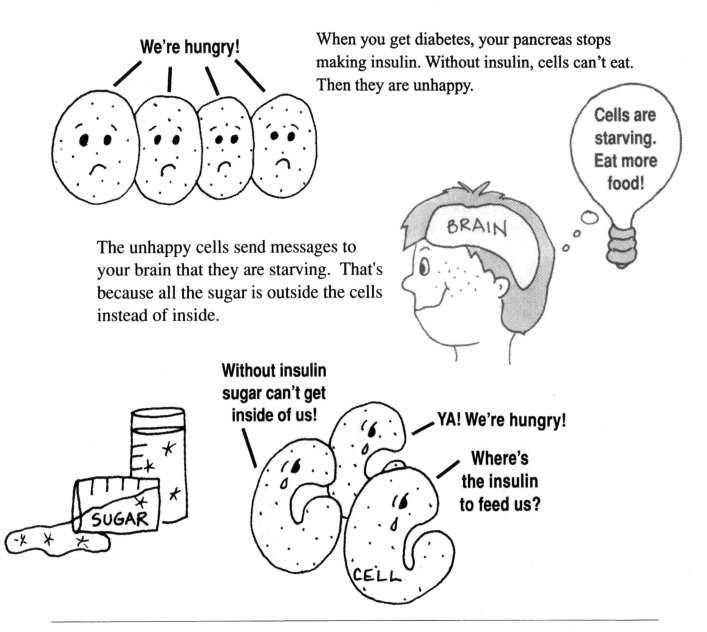

We're hungry!

When you get diabetes, your pancreas stops making insulin. Without insulin, cells can't eat. Then they are unhappy.

Cells are starving. Eat more food!

The unhappy cells send messages to your brain that they are starving. That's because all the sugar is outside the cells instead of inside.

BRAIN

Without insulin sugar can't get inside of us!

YA! We're hungry!

Where's the insulin to feed us?

SUGAR

CELL

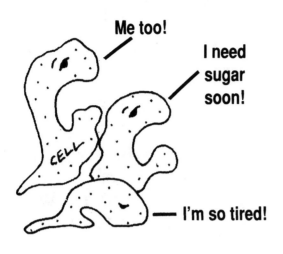

Me too!

I need sugar soon!

I'm so tired!

Your brain then sends a message to eat a lot of food. But your cells still can't eat because there isn't enough insulin to move sugar inside. Then you lose weight.

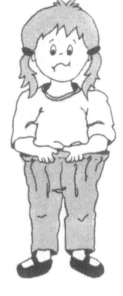

So the cells are starving, and you are hungry, tired, and losing weight.

The sugar from the food you eat can't get inside your cells and builds up in your blood. More and more sugar builds up until the extra sugar spills into your urine.

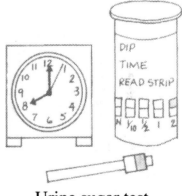

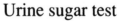

Urine sugar test

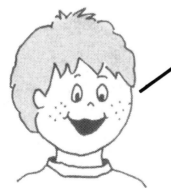

Then you have sugar in your urine! That's a sign of diabetes.

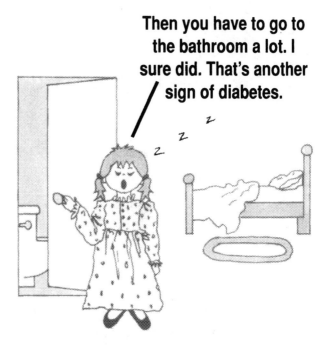

Thirsty all the time. That's another sign of diabetes.

When you have a lot of sugar in your urine, it pulls water from your body.

Then you have to go to the bathroom a lot. I sure did. That's another sign of diabetes.

And, because you lose a lot of water from your body, you can get very thirsty. Even though you might drink a whole lot, you still feel thirsty.

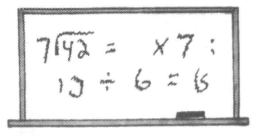

Signs of diabetes happen when your blood sugar is high. High blood sugar can also make things look blurry when you're trying to read or see things faraway.

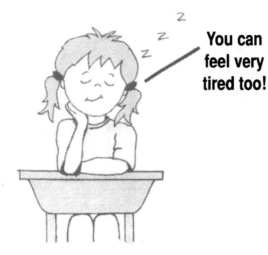

You can feel very tired too!

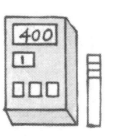

High blood sugar

Unscramble these signs of diabetes.

Write them here.

1. SLOE GIHTWE _____

2. OG OT ETH HBROATOM A OLT _____

_____

3. RHITSTY _____

4. DIRET _____

All the signs of diabetes, like being very thirsty, going to the bathroom a lot, blurred vision, and tiredness will go away after your body gets the insulin it needs. Without insulin, your body cannot grow. When you get the insulin you need, you will grow just fine.

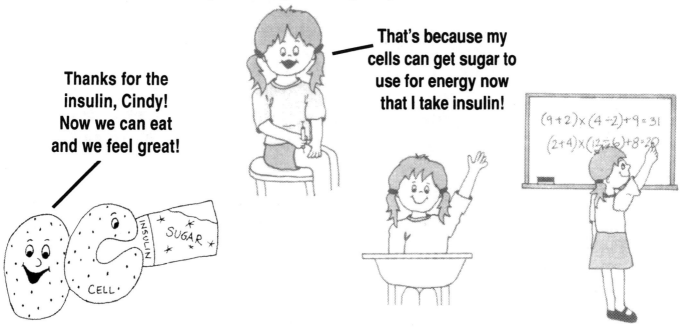

Thanks for the insulin, Cindy! Now we can eat and we feel great!

That's because my cells can get sugar to use for energy now that I take insulin!

Name _____ Date _____

Chapter 3.

All About Ketones

Ketones are made when you don't have enough insulin. When your cells are hungry, your body uses fat instead of sugar for energy. It's not healthy to use or "burn" fat for energy. Burning fat makes ketones. That is when you lose weight.

Ketones build up in your body and spill into your urine. They can act like a poison . . .

. . . and can make you very sick. Sometimes when people get diabetes the ketones make them vomit (throw up), and get very sleepy. They can make you feel like you can't breathe well.

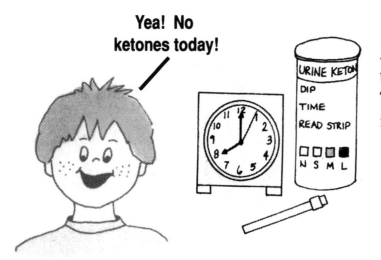

Yea! No ketones today!

A way to see if you have ketones is to urinate (pee) on a special strip. This strip will turn pink or purple if there are ketones in your urine.

* [Permission to use "Mr. Yuk" given by the Poison Control Center of Children's Hospital of Pittsburgh]

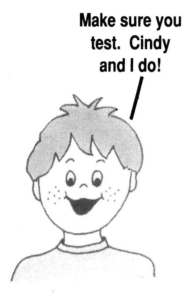

Make sure you test. Cindy and I do!

It's **very** important to check for ketones at these times:

1. In the morning before breakfast,

2. If blood sugars are high (over 240),

AND

3. When you are sick.

I have ketones this morning, Mom and Dad.

It's also very important to tell your parents or the person taking care of you if you have ketones.

When you have ketones, drink as much sugar-free soda or other diet drinks as you can.

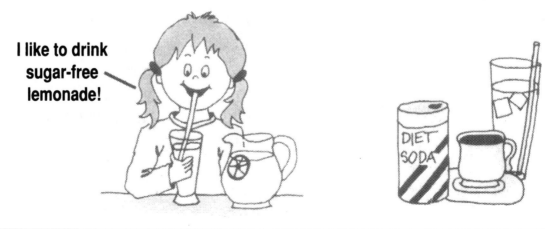

I like to drink sugar-free lemonade!

Fill in the missing word on each of these sentences about ketones.

SUGAR FREE SODA,   STRIP,   PARENTS,
SICK,   FAT,   SICK,   BEFORE,   HIGH

1. Burning _____ makes ketones.

2. Ketones can make you very _____.

3. You can see if you have ketones by urinating (peeing)
   on a special _____.

4. You should check for ketones:

   In the morning _____ breakfast.

   If blood sugars are _____.

   AND when you are _____.

5. Tell your _____ if you have ketones.

6. If you have ketones you

   should drink _____.

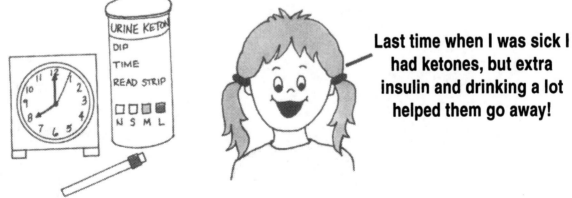

Last time when I was sick I
had ketones, but extra
insulin and drinking a lot
helped them go away!

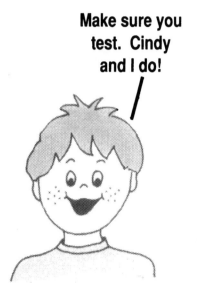

Make sure you test. Cindy and I do!

It's **very** important to check for ketones at these times:

1. In the morning before breakfast,

2. If blood sugars are high (over 240),

AND

3. When you are sick.

It's also very important to tell your parents or the person taking care of you if you have ketones.

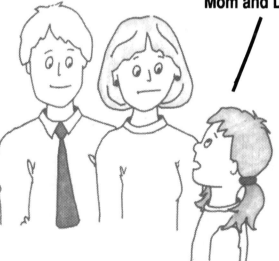

I have ketones this morning, Mom and Dad.

When you have ketones, drink as much sugar-free soda or other diet drinks as you can.

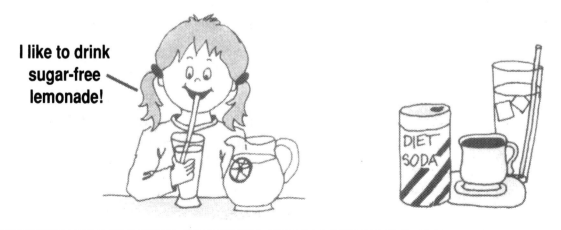

I like to drink sugar-free lemonade!

Fill in the missing word on each of these sentences about ketones.

SUGAR FREE SODA,   STRIP,   PARENTS,
SICK,   FAT,   SICK,   BEFORE,   HIGH

1. Burning _____ makes ketones.

2. Ketones can make you very _____.

3. You can see if you have ketones by urinating (peeing)
   on a special _____.

4. You should check for ketones:

    In the morning_____ breakfast.

    If blood sugars are _____.

    AND when you are _____.

5. Tell your _____ if you have ketones.

6. If you have ketones you

    should drink _____.

Last time when I was sick I
had ketones, but extra
insulin and drinking a lot
helped them go away!

Name _____ Date _____

Chapter 4.

Out of Balance: What Do I Do?

When you eat, your food travels to your stomach where it is turned into sugar. The sugar goes into your blood, and insulin helps it get into your cells. Cells use the sugar for energy!

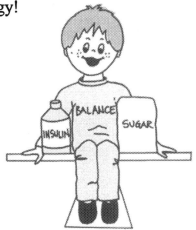

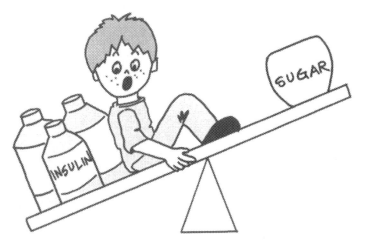

It is important to have a balance between how much sugar and insulin are in your blood.

If you don't have diabetes, when you eat, your pancreas makes insulin. This keeps blood sugar level in balance.

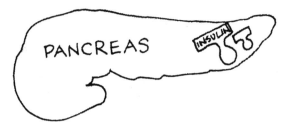

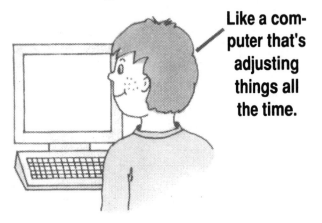

Like a computer that's adjusting things all the time.

Normally when blood sugar goes up, the body makes more insulin! When blood sugar goes down, the body makes less insulin.

Connect these sentences with the right ending.

1. The stomach's job is to turn food into   **cells.**

2. Insulin helps sugar get into   **insulin.**

3. Normally, when blood sugar goes up, the body makes   **sugar.**

When you have diabetes, your body can't make insulin. When you take insulin with a syringe, your body can't add more or make less.

Sometimes blood sugar can go out of balance. Your blood sugar might go too high or too low. People who have diabetes have to pay attention to their blood sugar balance every day.

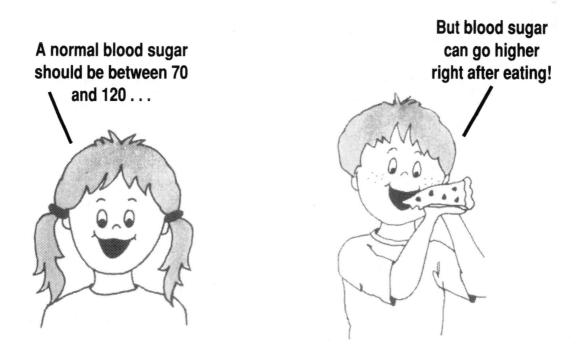

A normal blood sugar should be between 70 and 120 . . .

But blood sugar can go higher right after eating!

High blood sugar: What should I do?

A high blood sugar might happen if you:

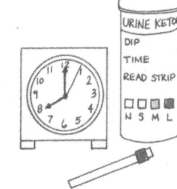

Sometimes I don't know why my blood sugar goes high!

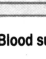

- eat too much food

- eat or drink sweet foods

- are sick

- are less active than usual (couch potato)

- don't take enough insulin.

And sometimes a high blood sugar can happen without a reason. When it does, write it down in your daily record book.

When you are high . . .

1. **Check your blood for sugar and your urine for ketones if blood sugar is over 240.**

   If you have any signs of urinating (peeing) a lot, thirst, blurry vision, or are tired, your blood sugar might be too high. Your body might be making ketones.

2. **Tell an adult if you don't feel well.**

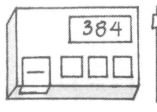

Blood sugar

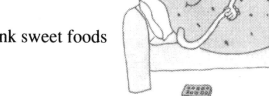

Urine ketones

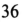

Connect these sentences with the right ending.

1. The stomach's job is to turn food into   **cells.**

2. Insulin helps sugar get into   **insulin.**

3. Normally, when blood sugar goes up, the body makes   **sugar.**

When you have diabetes, your body can't make insulin. When you take insulin with a syringe, your body can't add more or make less.

Sometimes blood sugar can go out of balance. Your blood sugar might go too high or too low. People who have diabetes have to pay attention to their blood sugar balance every day.

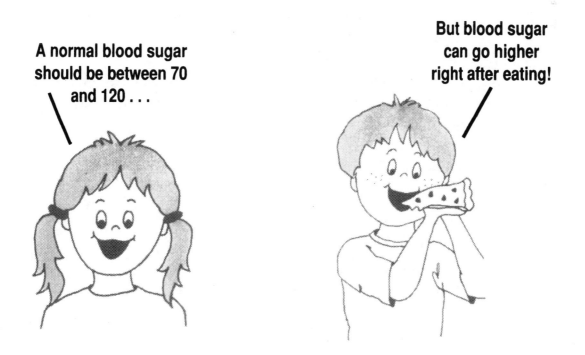

A normal blood sugar should be between 70 and 120 . . .

But blood sugar can go higher right after eating!

High blood sugar: What should I do?

A high blood sugar might happen if you:

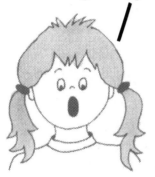

Sometimes I don't know why my blood sugar goes high!

- eat too much food

- eat or drink sweet foods

- are sick

- are less active than usual (couch potato)

- don't take enough insulin.

And sometimes a high blood sugar can happen without a reason. When it does, write it down in your daily record book.

When you are high . . .

1. **Check your blood for sugar and your urine for ketones if blood sugar is over 240.**

    If you have any signs of urinating (peeing) a lot, thirst, blurry vision, or are tired, your blood sugar might be too high. Your body might be making ketones.

2. **Tell an adult if you don't feel well.**

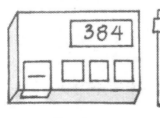

Blood sugar

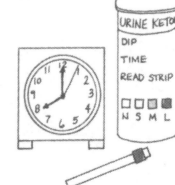

Urine ketones

If your blood sugar is very high or high at the same time every day, you may need to have a change in the amount of insulin you take.

If your blood sugar is a little high and you don't have ketones, exercise may help to bring down the high blood sugar.

But if you have ketones and you exercise, your body can make even more ketones! Then you might feel real sick! Ugh!

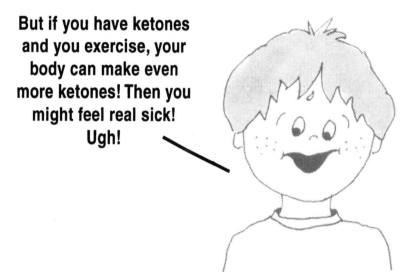

Have your doctor write in the number that is too high for you to exercise. _____

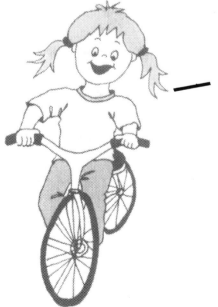

Last time I had high blood sugar, I rode my bike and my blood sugar came right down!

Answer these questions.

1. What are two things you should do if your blood sugar is high?

    (1)_____

    (2) _____

2. If you're feeling thirsty and tired, what might be happening to your blood sugar?

    _____

    _____

3. Normally, blood sugar before eating is between

        a. 40 and 70

        b. 70 and 120

        c. 120 and 200

        d. 200 and 300

4. Blood sugar usually goes up right after eating.   True   False

5. Exercise is a good way to get high blood sugar down when you don't have ketones.   True   False

6. You should not exercise if you have ketones.   True   False

Name _____ Date _____

Chapter 5.

Low Blood Sugar

When the balance between insulin, food, and exercise is upset, blood sugar can go too high (see Chapter 4) or too low.

A low blood sugar might happen if:

- You skip a meal or snack.

- A meal or snack is late.

- You don't eat enough.

- You are or have been exercising a lot.

- You are getting more insulin than your body needs.

Most often, when a low blood sugar happens, your body will give you warning signs. You might have strong signs or you might not even be able to tell you are low.

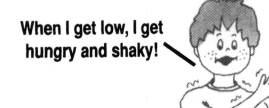

When I get low, I get hungry and shaky!

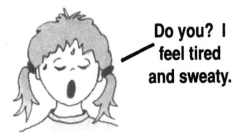

Do you? I feel tired and sweaty.

When you feel these signs, your body is telling you that you need more sugar in your blood.

Here are some signs of low blood sugar.
If you have had a low blood sugar, you may have felt some of these signs.

Circle the ways *you* felt.

    Shaky

    Sweaty

    Sleepy

    Tired

    Confused

    Like you can't think

    Weak

    Hungry

    Have a headache

    Dizzy

    Grouchy

    Cold

    Heart beating fast

    Have a nightmare (at night)

    Restless sleep (at night)

    Crying for no reason

When you feel signs of low blood sugar what you need to do very quickly is:

1. Eat or drink something sweet right away, **AND**

2. Tell someone you are feeling like your sugar is low, **AND**

I always tell my
teacher and my mom.

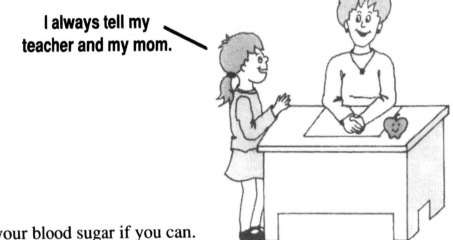

3. Test your blood sugar if you can.

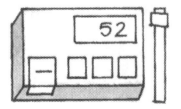

What should you eat or drink?

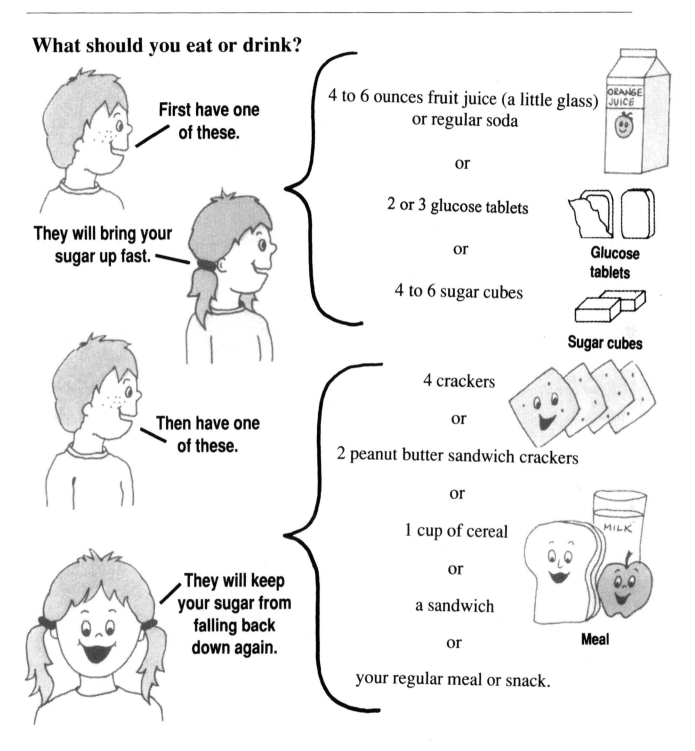

First have one of these.

They will bring your sugar up fast.

4 to 6 ounces fruit juice (a little glass) or regular soda

or

2 or 3 glucose tablets

or

4 to 6 sugar cubes

Glucose tablets

Sugar cubes

Then have one of these.

They will keep your sugar from falling back down again.

4 crackers

or

2 peanut butter sandwich crackers

or

1 cup of cereal

or

a sandwich

or

your regular meal or snack.

Meal

If you aren't feeling better in about 10 minutes, test your blood again (if you can), and eat and drink more if your sugar is still low.

Sometimes a friend can help—if they know what to do!

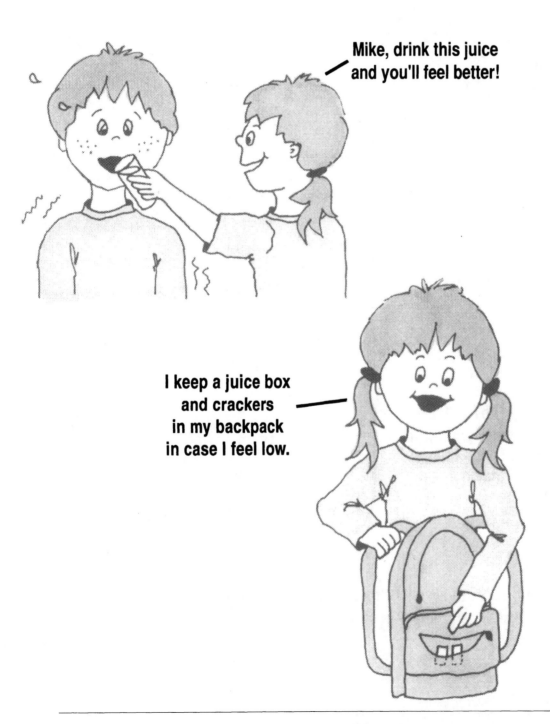

Mike, drink this juice and you'll feel better!

I keep a juice box and crackers in my backpack in case I feel low.

Circle the food that should be used to treat a low blood sugar. Draw an X through the foods that are NOT used to treat low blood sugar.

Diet soda	Coke	Water	Orange juice
Glucose tablet	Celery	Crackers	Sugar cube
Cheese crackers	Sandwich	Peanut butter crackers	
Grape jelly	Sugar-free gelatin		Raisins

In each box draw a picture of a person with the sign of low blood sugar.

Shaky	Sweaty	Sleepy	Hungry	Grouchy

Connect the signs on the left with high or low blood sugar.

Thirsty
Shaky   **High**
Sweaty
Nightmares
Urinating a lot   **Low**
Confused
Grouchy

It is very important to have some kind of sugar with you all the time in case you need it.

Draw a picture of the places you will keep your sugar.
Going to and from school. (Keep it in your pocket, purse, or backpack.)
During gym, recess, or sports. (Keep it in a pocket, helmet, tucked in your sock, or with your teacher or coach.)
On field trips or vacations. (Keep it in your pocket, purse, in the car or bus or give it to an adult who will be with you.)
When playing outside, biking, or exercising. (Keep it in your pocket, taped to your bike, in a back pack.)

Fill in the lines below.

When I do these activities:

_____

_____

_____

I will keep my sugar in these places:

_____

_____

_____

Sometimes the feelings of low blood sugar can be confused with other feelings, such as being scared or the way you feel after exercise. If you aren't sure if you are low, test your blood.

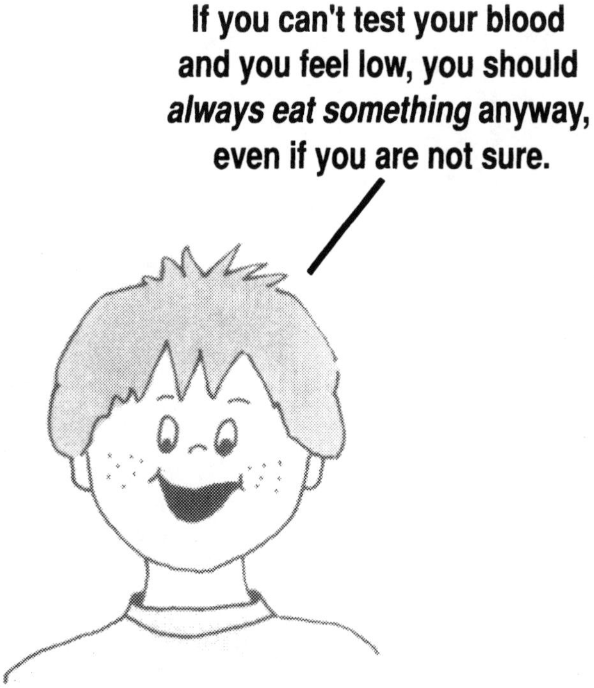

If you can't test your blood and you feel low, you should *always eat something* anyway, even if you are not sure.

What should you do if you feel you might be low, but you aren't sure?

_____

What kinds of foods would you eat or drink?

_____

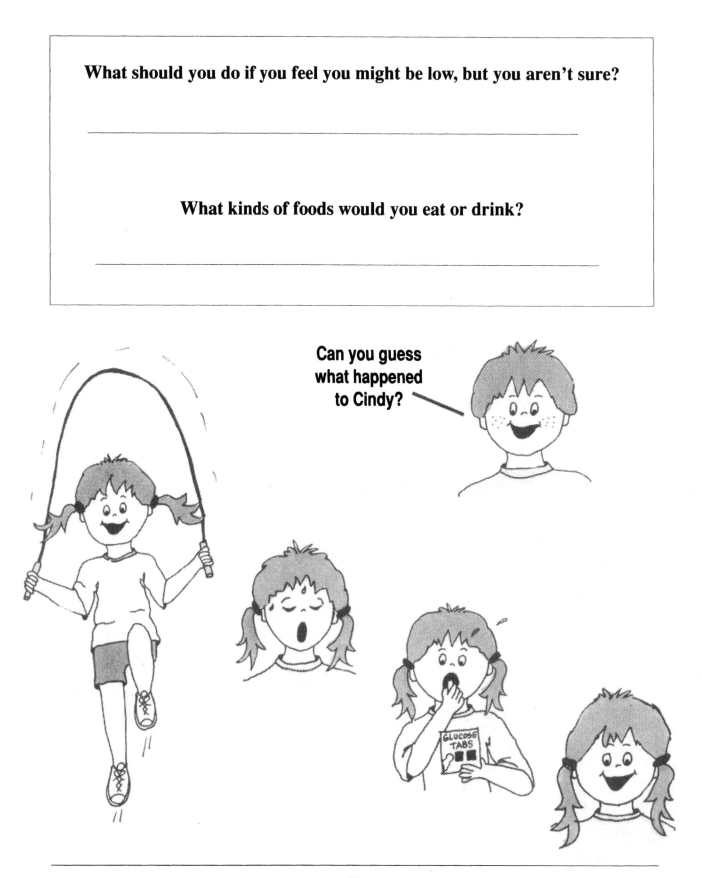

Can you guess
what happened
to Cindy?

Name _____ Date _____

Chapter 6.

Taking Insulin

There are many different kinds of insulin. Some insulin types work fast and others work slow. Your doctor will decide which insulin is best for you. Most children with diabetes take two kinds of insulin mixed together.

I take both NPH and Regular insulins.

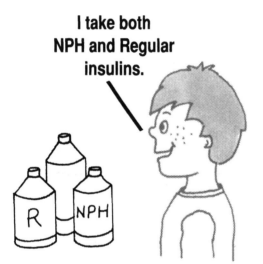

One kind of insulin, called Regular, looks like clear water and works very fast. It begins to work in about a half hour after you take it and works hard for about 3 hours.

Other kinds are called NPH or Lente and look cloudy in the bottle when you mix them. They work slowly, over a whole day, and work hardest about 8 hours after they're taken. Your doctor will decide which kind you will take.

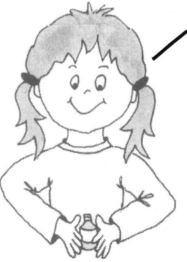

Don't forget to mix insulin before you use it. I roll the bottle in my hands to mix it up.

Connect the column on the left with the right kind of insulin.

Works slowly.

Cloudy.

REGULAR

Begins in 1/2 hour.

Works fast.

NPH or LENTE

Clear.

Works hardest in 8 hours.

Insulin is measured in units. The lines on your syringe mark the units. Your nurse will show you how to pull insulin into the syringe.

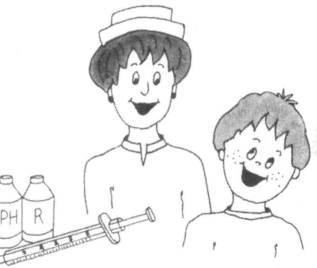

12 units. That's *exactly* right!

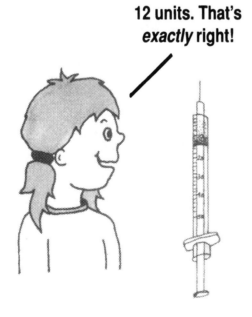

It is **very, very important** to make sure you have the right amount of insulin. If you make a mistake when you are pulling up your insulin, it is important to squirt it out and start all over. If you take the wrong dose, your blood sugar could go too high or too low.

Also, check your syringe for air bubbles. If you have a big, fat air bubble, you won't be getting the right amount of insulin. It's a good idea to have someone else check your syringe before you take your insulin just to make sure everything is OK.

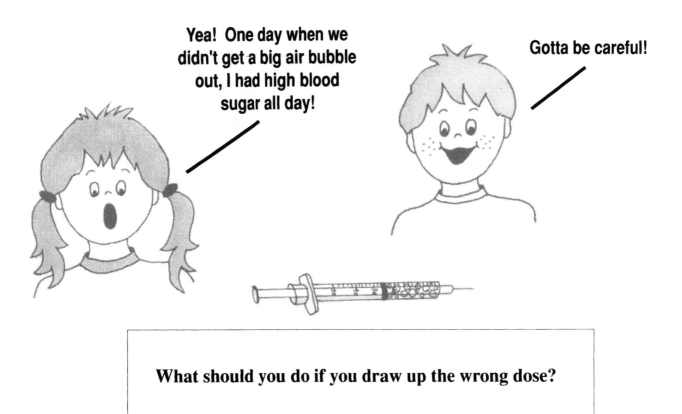

What should you do if you draw up the wrong dose?

_____

_____

You can take insulin in your arms, legs, tummy, and hips. Your doctor or nurse will tell you where your best spots are. It is important to give your insulin in a different spot every day. It works at different speeds at each spot. If the spot where you give your insulin gets puffy or lumpy, the insulin may not work as well as it should. Move to a new spot!

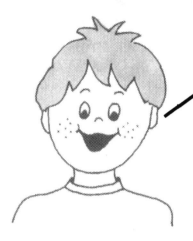

Pick a new spot everyday! See where the best spots are on the drawings below. I take mine in my arms in the the morning, tummy at dinner and legs at bedtime.

Make sure you pinch up the spot. If you look for a spot where you can pinch a little fat, you will be sure you aren't taking your insulin in your muscle. Insulin might work faster if you put it in your muscle instead of fat.

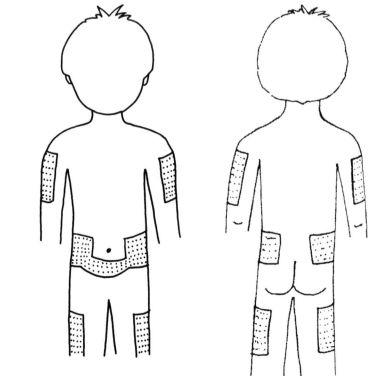

Put the needle straight into the pinched up spot. You can learn to
pinch up your arms yourself.

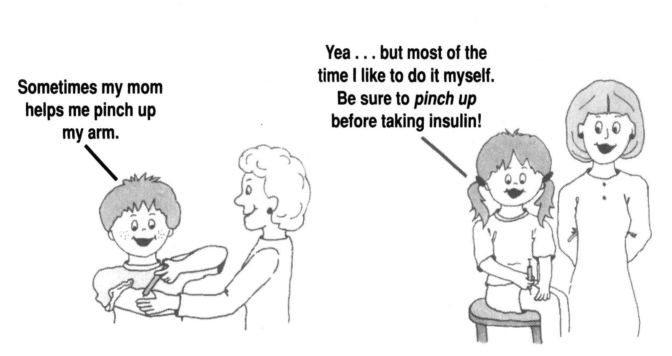

Draw an X on each of the places where you can take your insulin.

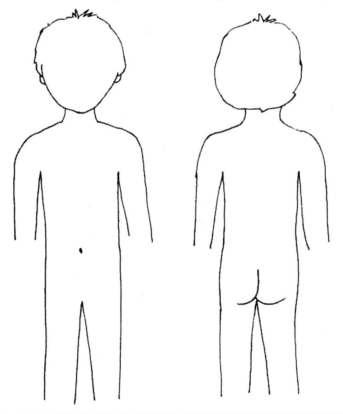

Taking Insulin Crossword Puzzle

Across

2. You don't want these in your syringe.

4. This goes into the syringe.

7. Always take your insulin in different _ _ _ _ _.

8. When you take two kinds of insulin, you learn to _ _ _.

9. The fast insulin that looks like water.

Down

1. Pinch up so you don't get your insulin in a _ _ _ _ _ _.

3. One kind of cloudy, slow insulin.

5. Insulin is measured in these.

6. Do this to your fat when you give your insulin.

7. You pull your insulin into this.

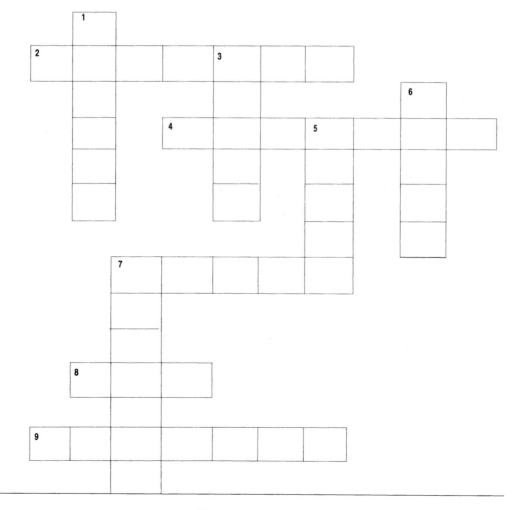

Name _____ Date _____

Chapter 7.

Testing Blood and Urine

One way to help balance your blood sugar is to do blood testing. You can only balance your blood sugar with exercise and food, if you know what your blood sugar level is.

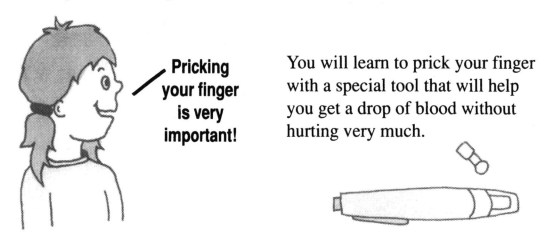

Pricking your finger is very important!

You will learn to prick your finger with a special tool that will help you get a drop of blood without hurting very much.

There are many different ways to test your blood. Your doctor or nurse will help you and your parents decide which is the best way for you.

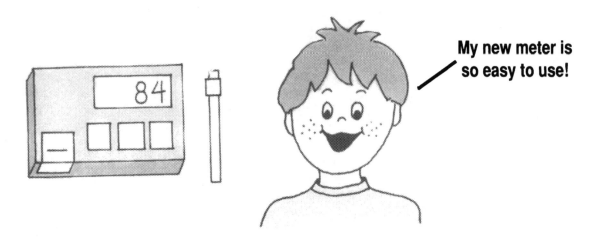

My new meter is so easy to use!

How to test blood sugar . . .

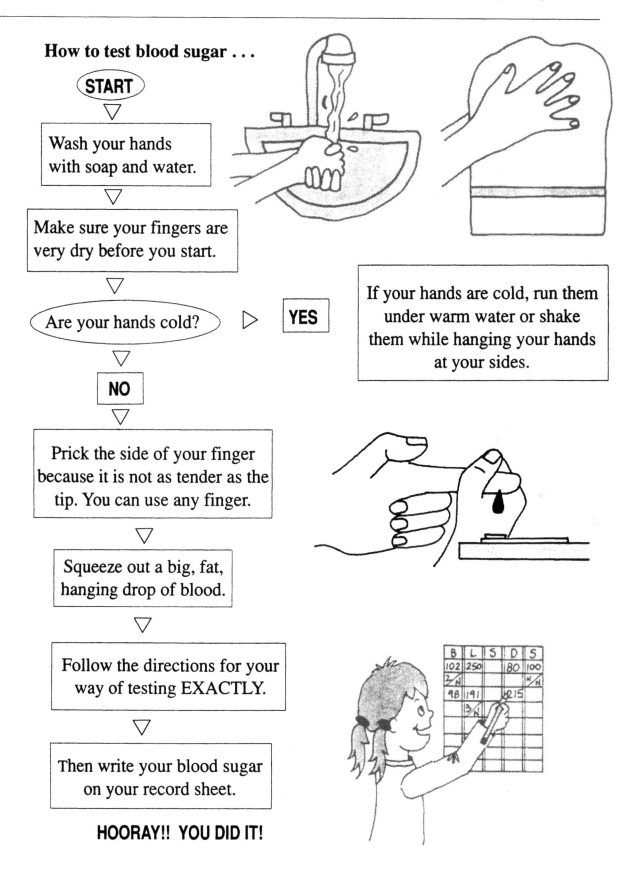

START

Wash your hands with soap and water.

Make sure your fingers are very dry before you start.

Are your hands cold?

▷ **YES**

NO

If your hands are cold, run them under warm water or shake them while hanging your hands at your sides.

Prick the side of your finger because it is not as tender as the tip. You can use any finger.

Squeeze out a big, fat, hanging drop of blood.

Follow the directions for your way of testing EXACTLY.

Then write your blood sugar on your record sheet.

HOORAY!! YOU DID IT!

How often to test . . .

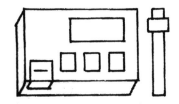

It is important to test often. Most children test their blood 3, 4 or more times every day. Your doctor, nurse, or parents will tell you how often and at what times to do it.

The usual times to test are before breakfast, lunch, dinner and bedtime snack. Sometimes you may even need to test during the night.

Test *before* meals because after you eat blood sugar goes up.

Have your doctor or nurse write your times to test here:

_____

You may need to test your blood sugar between your usual times to see if it is too high or too low.

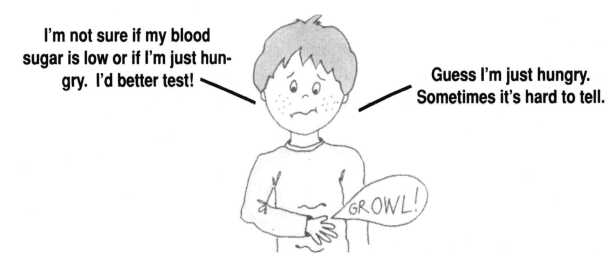

I'm not sure if my blood sugar is low or if I'm just hungry. I'd better test!

Guess I'm just hungry. Sometimes it's hard to tell.

Circle the times you will usually test your blood at home.

Before breakfast   After breakfast   Before lunch   After lunch

Before dinner   After dinner   Before snack   During the night

When I'm not feeling good

Don't forget to write your tests in your daily record book. This will help your doctors, nurses, and parents decide how much insulin you need. You will only be able to keep in balance if you have it all written down. It's also smart to write food and exercise in your book if it helps to explain a high or low blood sugar.

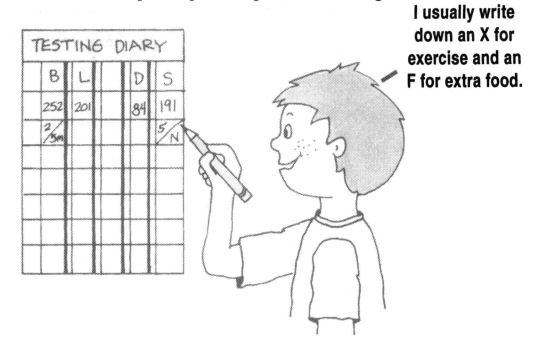

I usually write down an X for exercise and an F for extra food.

Name _____ Date _____

Chapter 8.

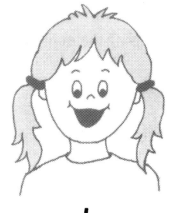

Healthy Eating

We should eat food that is good for our bodies. Children need food to grow and for energy. It is especially important for people with diabetes to have healthy eating habits.

**F A T . . . No way!
Not if you eat right!**

The 3 R's of healthy eating are:
- the **Right** **F**oods
- in the **Right** **A**mounts
- at the **Right** **T**imes.

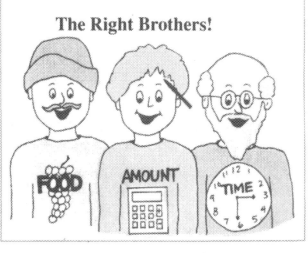

**The Right Brothers
will help you keep
the balance.**

A dietitian is someone who helps with your meal plan. Your dietitian will explain all about your meal plan.

Keeping a balance between food, exercise, and insulin works best when you stay on a schedule.

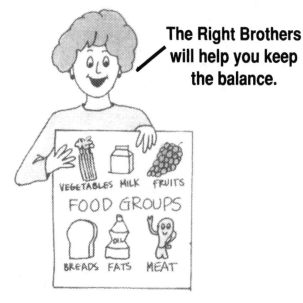

What are the "Right Foods"?

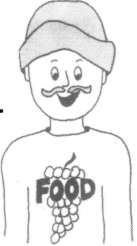

Because some food makes blood sugar levels go higher than other foods, you will be given a plan for balancing your meals. The plan will let you pick from these groups.

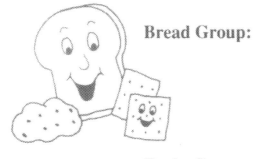

Bread Group:

Easy for your body to turn into sugar.

Includes: bread, crackers, cereal, potatoes, rice, peas, corn, pasta

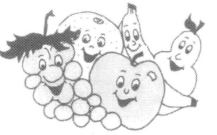

Fruit Group:

Easy for your body to turn into sugar.

Includes: apples, fruit juice, bananas, raisins, oranges

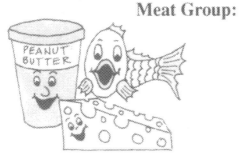

Meat Group:

Turns into sugar more slowly.

Includes: chicken, cheese, peanut butter, eggs, beef, fish

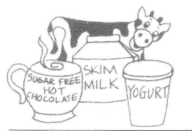

Milk Group:

Turns into sugar more easily than the meat group but not as easy as bread and fruit.

Includes: low-fat white milk, yogurt

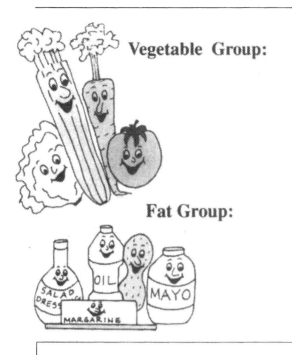

Vegetable Group: Usually doesn't change blood sugar levels much.

Includes: *lettuce, green and yellow string beans, broccoli, carrots, tomatoes*

Fat Group: Doesn't change blood sugar much.

Includes: *margarine, nuts, oil, olives, salad dressing*

List these foods under the food group they belong in.

Bananas	Cheese	Eggs	Carrots	Crackers
Nuts	Lettuce	Peas	Peanut butter	Cereal
Milk	Apples	Yogurt	Salad dressing	

Bread	Fruit	Meat	Milk	Vegetable	Fat

When you have diabetes, you take your insulin in a syringe. Your body can't make more if you need it, and you can't shut it off if you have too much.

Eating sweet foods (like cake, pie, or candy) between meals, or eating a lot of them with a meal can send blood sugar too high. Insulin can't balance it.

When you have a sweet food, such as at a birthday party or after a soccer game, it is smart to plan ahead so you can balance it with extra insulin or exercise.

I like to eat cake at birthday parties.

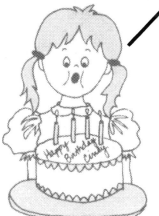

After a soccer game, I like to eat ice cream.

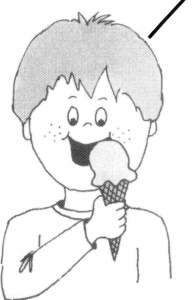

When you plan to have a sweet, one smart time to have it might be when you plan to be very active. Another time might be when your blood sugar level is low. Your dietitian will tell you how to work candy or desserts into your meal plan.

We all should watch how much and what kinds of fat we eat. This is even more important for people who have diabetes. Certain kinds of fat (BAD fats called saturated fat and cholesterol) can clog up blood vessels.

Cholesterol is found in butter, fatty meats, eggs, and cheese.

Saturated fats are found in the same foods as cholesterol but also in some oils such as palm and coconut oil.

Good fats are called unsaturated fats and are in corn oil, olive oil, and vegetable oil.

What is the **Right Amount** of food?

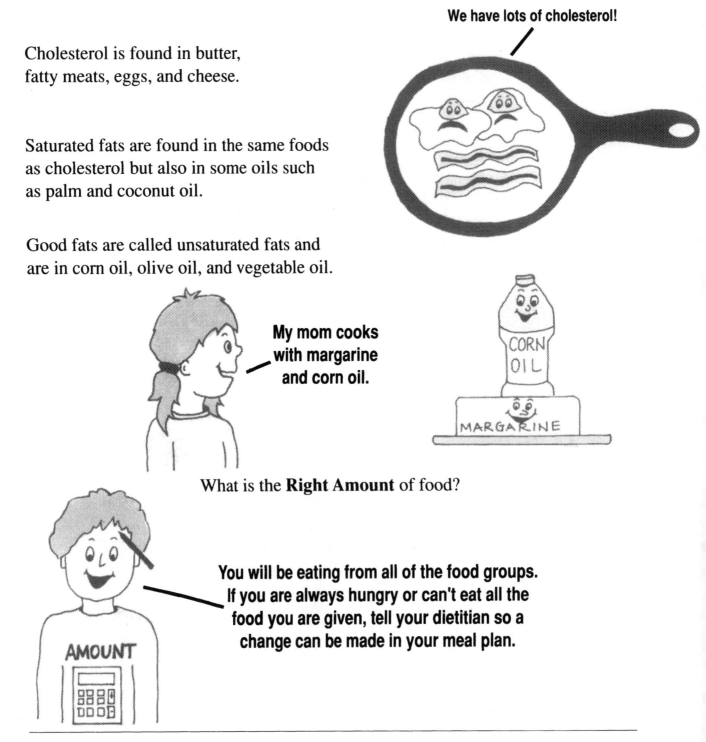

We have lots of cholesterol!

My mom cooks with margarine and corn oil.

CORN OIL

MARGARINE

AMOUNT

You will be eating from all of the food groups. If you are always hungry or can't eat all the food you are given, tell your dietitian so a change can be made in your meal plan.

When you have been exercising and are extra hungry, you will need more food at meal times. Just make sure you eat the extra food from all food groups.

What is the **Right Time** to eat?

Most children who must take insulin eat breakfast, lunch, afternoon snack, dinner, and bedtime snack. It is important to stay on schedule so meals and snacks can balance insulin.

If lunch is more than 4 hours after breakfast, you may need a morning snack.

If you stay within 1 hour of your normal schedule for meals and snacks, your blood sugar balance should be OK.

Write down the times of your normal schedule. You may not do all of these things all of the time. If not, leave it blank.

Activity	Time
Wake up	_____
Test blood and urine	_____
Take insulin	_____
Eat breakfast	_____
Morning snack	_____
Test blood	_____
Take insulin	_____
Eat lunch	_____
Afternoon snack	_____
Test blood	_____
Take insulin	_____
Eat dinner	_____
Test blood	_____
Eat bedtime snack	_____
Take insulin	_____

Your schedule is probably a little bit different from mine.

That's because my bus comes earlier than yours.

Yeah, plus I have soccer practice after school.

If you are extra hungry at meal time and want to eat more, what should you eat?

_____

_____

You should try to keep your meals and snacks within _____ (how much time) of your normal schedule.

Name _____ Date _____

Chapter 9.

Exercise Is Fun!

Exercise is fun and healthy for almost everyone.

Circle the kinds of exercise you do!

Running	Biking	Swimming	Football	Baseball	Softball
Soccer	Walking	Hiking	Track	Wrestling	Dance
Gynmastics		Skiing	Kickball	Hockey	

Other _____

Exercise keeps your body fit and can be fun. Team sports help people have fun together. When you exercise you will need to know how to keep your blood sugar balanced.

When you are exercising, your muscles use more sugar from your blood. So when you exercise, you MUST EAT MORE food to put back the sugar your muscles used.

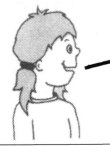

Always carry a snack with you. I like raisins and cheese crackers.

If you plan to exercise after a meal, you will need to eat more at the meal. Other times you may need to eat a snack before exercise. Here are some ideas for snack foods you can eat before you exercise.

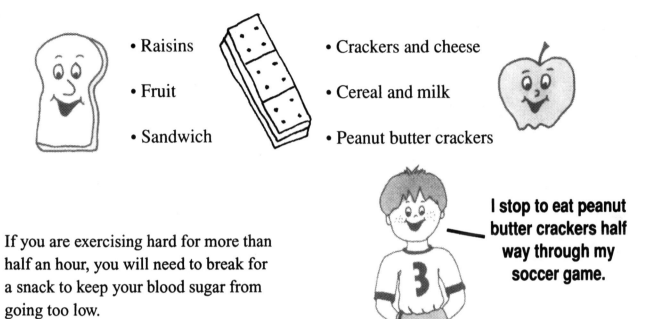

- Raisins

- Fruit

- Sandwich

- Crackers and cheese

- Cereal and milk

- Peanut butter crackers

I stop to eat peanut butter crackers half way through my soccer game.

If you are exercising hard for more than half an hour, you will need to break for a snack to keep your blood sugar from going too low.

If you are planning to do a lot of exercise, like hiking or skiing all day, your doctor might tell you to also take less insulin that day.

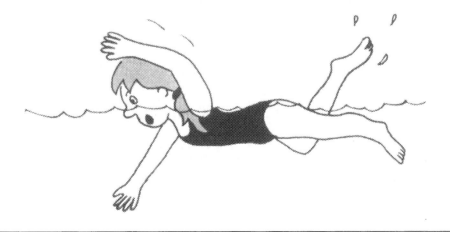

Some things you do don't burn much sugar because your muscles don't work much.

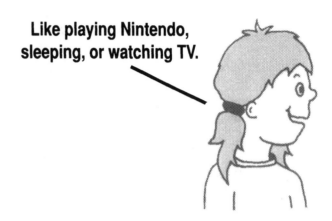

Like playing Nintendo, sleeping, or watching TV.

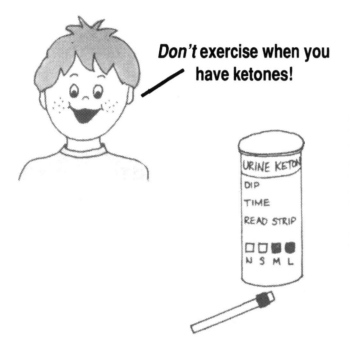

***Don't* exercise when you have ketones!**

Most of the time, blood sugar goes down when you exercise. But, if you don't have *enough* insulin when you exercise, you can break down fat. Then blood sugar may go up instead of down! Ketones can also increase.

What is the number that is too high for you to exercise? _____ (See page 37.)

Circle the exercises that help muscles use sugar quickly.

Walking	Biking	Swimming	Playing Nintendo	Baseball
Kickball	Hockey	Basketball	Running	Watching TV
Tennis	Soccer	Sleeping	Talking on phone	

My Pledge of Safety

Fill in the blanks.

I promise I will always keep _____ with
(Kind of sugar.)

me in my _____ when I _____.
(Place where you'll carry it.)　　　　　　　　　　　(Kind of exercise you do.)

Remember! Always have some fast sugar with you while you are exercising.

Be ready to treat a low blood sugar if it happens. Have fun by keeping it safe!

Name _____ Date _____

Chapter 10.

Balancing It All

Keeping the balance—that's the hard part!

When you have diabetes, three things must be balanced to keep blood sugar normal.

Circle the 3 things that must stay in balance to keep blood sugars normal.

Insulin   Ketones   Exercise   Thirst   Food

If you don't remember, go back to Chapter 4 to find the answers.

When any one of these things goes out of balance, your blood sugar can go too high or too low.

In this book we will call a high blood sugar anything over 180 and a low blood sugar anything under 70. Your doctor might give you different numbers that are just right for you.

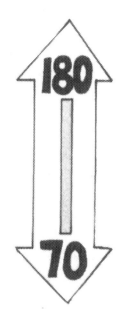

Anything between 70 and 180 is OK.
A blood sugar of around 100 is normal.

Circle the meters with blood sugars that are right for you.

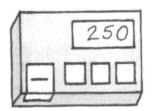
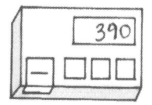
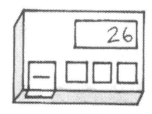

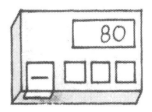
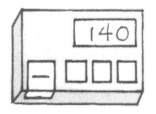
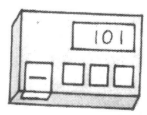

Here is a chart of what you will need to think about every day. On one side are the things that can cause your blood sugar to go up and on the other side, things that can cause blood sugar to go down. When something is happening on one side, you will need to pick something on the other side to balance it.

Makes blood sugar go UP	**Makes blood sugar go DOWN**
Not enough insulin	Too much insulin
Too much food or sweet foods	Not enough food
Stress, cold, flu, feeling upset	Exercise

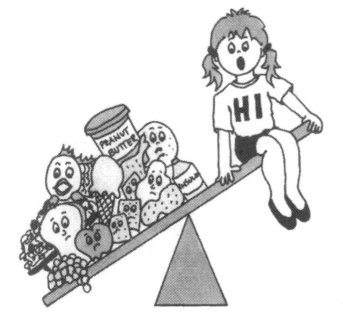
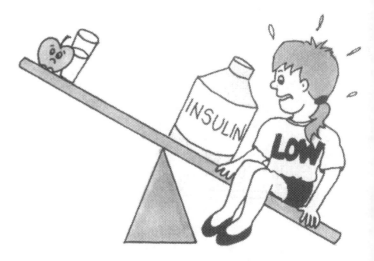

Here are some things that could happen to make blood sugar go up or down.

• Read the problem.

• Then decide if that problem would make blood sugars go up or down.

• Write down what you could do to balance blood sugar again.

Example:

1. Cindy has a bad cold.

This would probably make her blood sugar go ___**UP**___ .

One thing Cindy could do to keep the balance might be to

___**TAKE MORE INSULIN**___ .

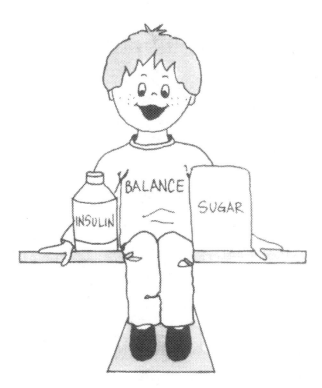

2. Mike is going to play softball.

This would probably make his blood sugar go _____.

One thing Mike could do to keep the balance might be to

_____.

3. Mike wants to have extra pizza at a party with his friends.

This would probably make his blood sugar go _____.

One thing he could do to keep the balance might be to

_____.

4. Some of Cindy's insulin leaked out when she took her insulin.

This would probably make her blood sugar go _____ .

One thing she could do to keep the balance might be to

_____ .

When you are all done, you can check
your answers on the next page.

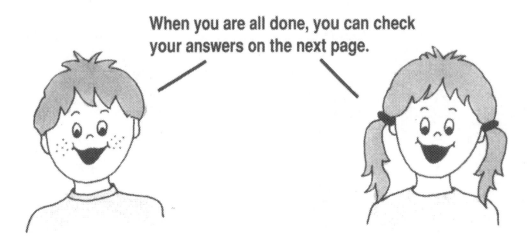

Answers

1. When anyone with diabetes is sick, his or her blood sugar level usually goes **up**. (Body cells need extra insulin when they're sick.)

   If Cindy is not eating much because she's sick, her blood sugar level may be okay. If her blood sugar is too high, Cindy might need to take more insulin. Cindy should not exercise if she's sick. (See Chapter 11, **When I'm Sick.**)

2. If Mike is going to be exercising, his blood sugar level will probably go **down** because his muscles will be using sugar.

   Mike should eat some peanut butter crackers before his game. If he plays hard, he should have juice and crackers between innings.

3. Mike knows that the extra food will probably cause his blood sugar to go **up**.

   If he can plan ahead, Mike and his parents might decide to give extra insulin. Mike also might be able to get some exercise after he eats to keep in balance.

4. Cindy knows that if she doesn't get all her insulin, her blood sugar will probably go **up**.

   She might try to get extra exercise (if she doesn't have ketones). Or she could eat a little bit less if she doesn't feel like eating much.

Keeping the balance isn't easy! Sometimes it's hard to keep on a schedule

The more you know about how to adjust insulin, the better you'll know how to keep in balance.

Sleeping late in the morning when you have diabetes just doesn't work! It messes up my blood sugars!

Staying on Schedule

Sometimes you may want to sleep more than one hour past your usual time to get up. One way to get the extra sleep is to get up on time, test, take your insulin, **eat**, and then go back to bed.

Sometimes you might try very hard to keep in balance and it just doesn't work.

Keep trying!! Sometimes you have to try different ways to see what works best for you.

In the summer most children with diabetes eat all
their meals and snacks later to keep in balance.

What is one good way to keep in balance and still sleep in the morning?

_____

_____

_____

Name _____ Date _____

Chapter 11.

When I'm Sick

When you have diabetes and get sick with a cold or flu, blood sugar can go out of balance. Most of the time when you're sick, blood sugar levels will go up. Ketones may be in your urine.

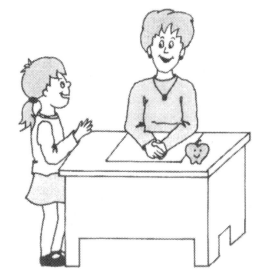

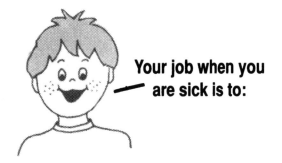

Your job when you are sick is to:

1. Tell someone (parent, teacher) that you aren't feeling well. Always tell someone if you vomit (throw up).

2. Test your blood sugar every 4 hours.

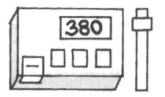

3. Check your urine for ketones, and tell your parents if the ketone strip is pink or purple. You will need to check every time you urinate (pee) as long as you are sick or until the ketones go away.

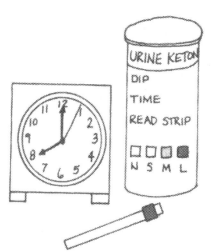

4. Drink as many sugar-free drinks as you can.

5. Rest! If you have ketones and you exercise, it can make more ketones.

6. Always take your insulin.

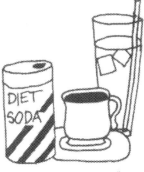

We're always here to help!

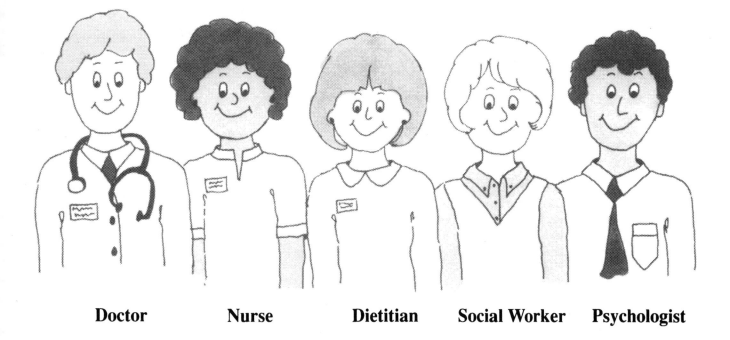

Doctor　　　Nurse　　　Dietitian　　Social Worker　Psychologist

When I'm Sick . . .
Crossword Puzzle

Down

1. Tell my parents if my urine test turns pink or __ __ __ __ __ __ .

3. __ __ __ __ __ sugar-free beverages.

4. I should test my __ __ __ __ __ sugar every four hours.

5. I check my urine for

__ __ __ __ __ __ __ .

Across

2. When I'm sick, my blood sugar will probably go __ __.

4. When I'm sick, my blood sugar can go out of __ __ __ __ __ __ __ .

6. I should always tell some if I __ __ __ __ __ .

7. When I'm sick I should __ __ __ __ .

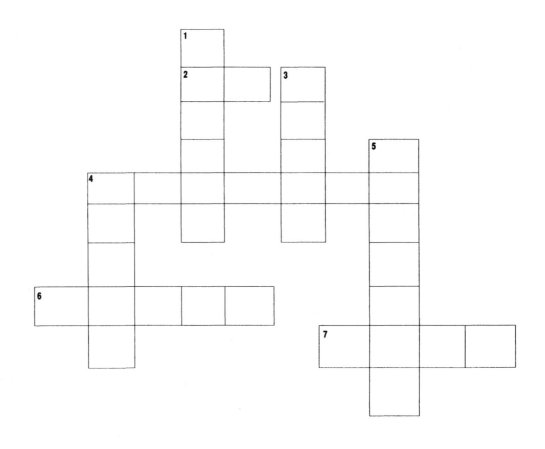

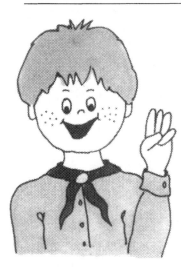

Name _____ Date _____

Chapter 12.

Party Time

Sometimes when parties or holidays come up, you may need to make some changes to keep blood sugar in balance. The very best way of keeping in balance is to plan ahead. Your nurse, dietitian, or doctor will be able to help you plan your day. You can take good care of your diabetes and still do all of the fun things you want to do.

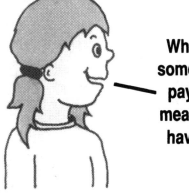

When I'm at a party, sometimes it's hard to pay attention to my meal plan. Mike and I have some tips that work for us.

Boy Scout cookout and award night.

Party Tips

1. Find out ahead of time if a meal will be served, what time, and what foods are planned.

2. Ask if there will be diet soda. If not, take some with you.

3. You may plan to have a sweet food at the party. (If you can, get some exercise later.) Ask your doctor or nurse if you will need to adjust insulin doses.

4. If you choose not to have a sweet food ask for some fresh fruit for dessert or bring your own.

Sleeping Over, Trips, and Vacations

Planning ahead is the key to being able to do all the things you want and still keep your blood sugar in balance.

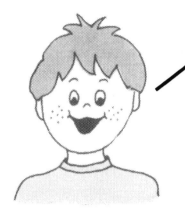

Cindy and I have more tips for travel . . .

1. Make sure somebody with you knows you have diabetes and can treat low blood sugar.

2. Talk to your doctor or nurse about what to do if you have a problem while you are away.

3. Take more supplies than you think you will need, such as insulin, syringes, and blood and urine testing equipment, in case yours gets lost. Make sure you have plenty of sugar in case you are low.

4. Always wear your identification (ID) bracelet or chain. (See chapter 15.)

5. Keep your insulin in a thermos or cool pack when you travel. Never let it get hot or frozen.

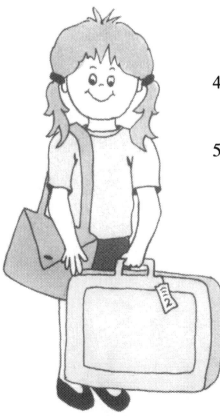

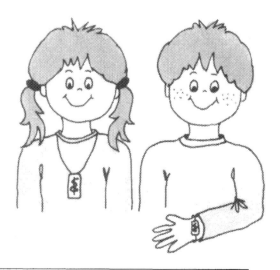

Answer these questions.

1. Where is a place you might go away from home?

   _____

2. Who might be with you who knows about low blood sugar?

   _____

3. What supplies might you take along?

   _____

4. Where will you keep your supplies?

   _____

5. How will you keep your insulin from getting too warm?

   _____

Have fun! But keep it safe!!

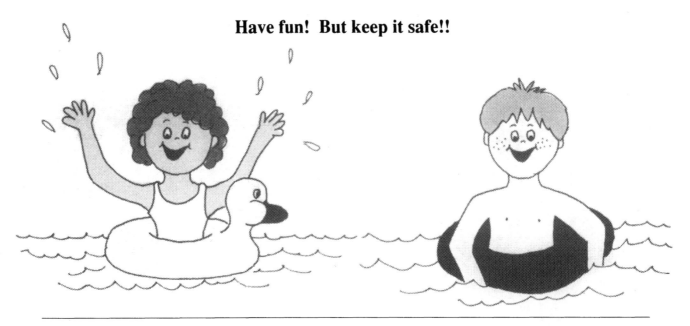

Name _____ Date _____

Chapter 13.

Diabetes in School

When you have diabetes, you, your parents, teachers, coaches, and others from your school should have a meeting to decide the best way to manage your diabetes while you are in school.

Together you will need to decide a plan for:

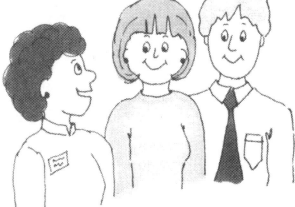

1. Managing your schedule.

If you need to have a snack in school, you will have to decide on the best time to eat it. Some children eat their snack in the classroom, while others go to the lunchroom or office.

On gym days, you may need to eat some crackers or a sandwich before gym. If gym is after breakfast or lunch, you can eat more at those meals.

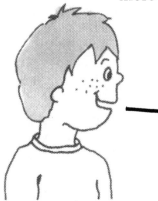

If you have a field trip or activity that might make lunch or snack late, tell someone and take sugar and crackers with you.

2. Low blood sugar.

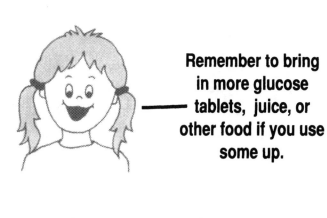

Remember to bring in more glucose tablets, juice, or other food if you use some up.

Some children pack what they call a "low box," which they keep in the teacher's desk. Pack glucose tablets, juice, or raisins and crackers. Keep a box in all your classrooms, the gym, with your coach, and in the library. If you feel your blood sugar is too low, you can eat something out of the box.

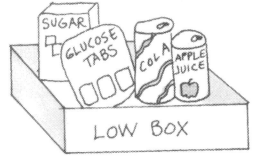

If you have a low blood sugar in school, ask your teacher if you can be excused from any test or report for about an hour or so after you feel better. The wait is to make sure you are able to think clearly.

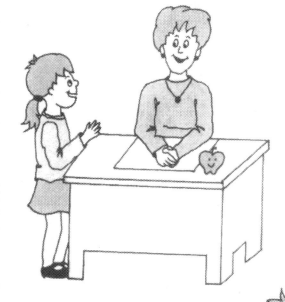

You need to:
1. Tell the teacher that you are feeling low;
2. Eat something sweet; and
3. Tell your parents when you get home.

3. High blood sugar.

If your blood sugar is running high, you may need to ask your teacher for extra trips to the water fountain or bathroom. A note from Mom or Dad to your teacher might help at these times.

Ask your parents for a note if you need one.

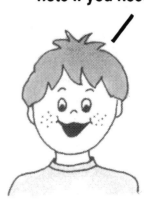

> *Dear Miss Beatle,*   *Tuesday*
> *   Mike's blood sugars are running high this morning. Please excuse him to the restroom as needed.*
> *   Thank you,*
> *   Marcia Adams*

4. Lunch room eating.

Sometimes it is hard to stick to your meal plan when you see other children eating fatty or sweet foods at lunch time.

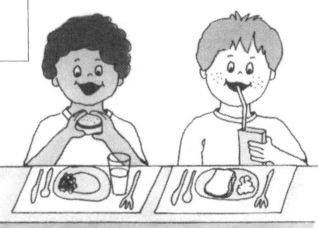

Pack a lunch that you really like. Choose not to "trade" away your healthy foods. You need them.

Bring home the menu so you can plan what you need at lunch time.

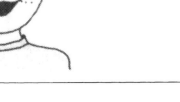

Most schools give out their menu a week or a month ahead of time. Show it to your parents so that together you can decide which meals to eat. Most schools will let you exchange a piece of fruit for the school dessert and have skim or low-fat milk if you ask.

5. *Classroom parties*.

If you know there is going to be a party in school at Halloween, Christmas, or Valentine's Day, you need to plan ahead. You may decide to eat some of the party foods for a special treat.

Most children keep a party box in the classroom or in their locker. Pack foods in your party box that you enjoy and that will be healthy for you to eat.

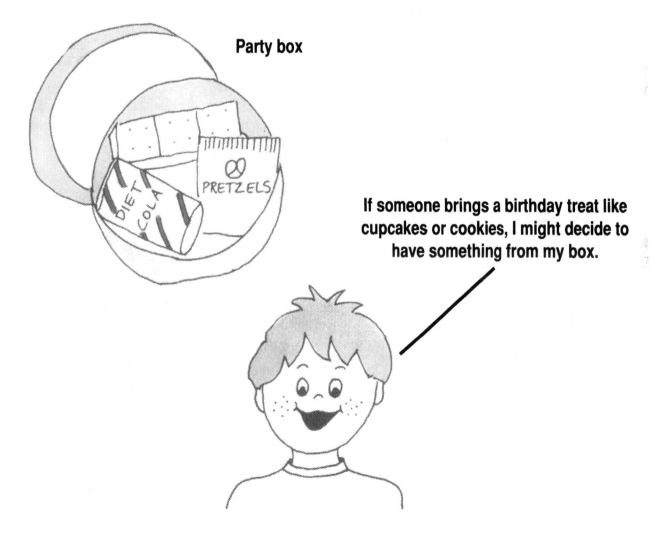

Party box

If someone brings a birthday treat like cupcakes or cookies, I might decide to have something from my box.

It's smart to make sure you have foods around that you can eat.

Ideas for your party box might be: Diet soda, pretzels, trail mix, peanuts, raisins, vanilla wafers, and animal crackers. Sometimes a friend might bring in a healthy food treat that you and everyone can eat.

What food items will you pack in your party box?

_____

_____

_____

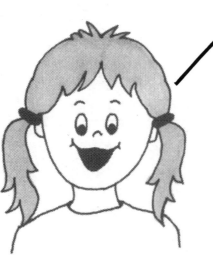

Tell your parents what foods you use so they can keep your party box supplied. And decide, with your teacher and parents, the best way to handle parties in school.

Name _____ Date _____

Chapter 14.

Keep It Safe

Since you are now using syringes and lancets, you have a very important job.

Your job is to keep yourself and other people safe.

Someone could get stuck by your needle or lancet if you aren't careful.

**Here are some rules for
keeping things safe.**

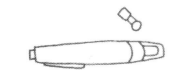

1. Be careful never to stick yourself or anyone else with a used needle or lancet.

- Reason: People can pass germs to each other when needles and lancets are shared.

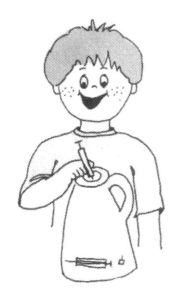

2. Put all your needles and lancets in an empty plastic milk jug for safety.

- Reason: Little children and others will not get stuck, and you can throw the needles away safely.

Connect the rules on the left with the correct reason on the right.

Don't prick yourself
   with a used needle.

People won't get stuck.

You can throw them
   safely in the garbage.

Safely throw out all syringes.

Put them in an empty
   plastic milk jug.

People can pass germs
   by sharing needles.

Name _____ Date _____

Chapter 15.

Managing on My Own

You are the only one who is with you all the time! So you will need to learn as much as you can about diabetes so you can take very good care of yourself.

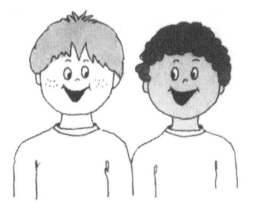

Sometimes friends like to learn about diabetes so they can help. Your best friends should know to give you sugar or juice if you have a low blood sugar.

Which friends do you think you'll tell about your diabetes?

_____

_____

_____

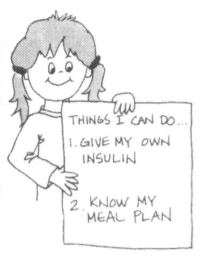

You will probably want to learn to give your own insulin and do your own blood tests so you can sleep overnight at a friend's house. (See Chapter 12.)

And you will need to know your own meal plan so you can make healthy choices at school, with friends, and when you play.

Many people can help you take care of yourself, like parents, brothers, sisters, grandparents, friends, your doctor, nurse, and dietitian.

Medical Identification (ID)

When you have diabetes, you always wear a tag or bracelet that says, "I have diabetes." Your doctor or nurse can tell your parents where to buy one.

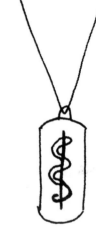

It is important to wear your ID all the time. When you are on your own (out riding your bike or playing), if you are hurt, or if you are in an accident, someone could find out from your ID that you have diabetes. Then you would get proper medical care.

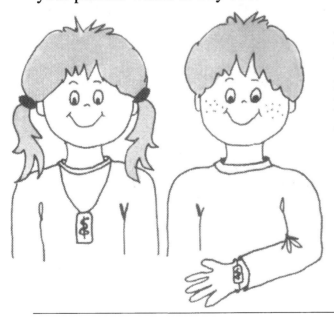

Tips for managing on your own.

1. The more you do for yourself, the more your parents may let you do. You will have shown your parents you are able to take good care of yourself.

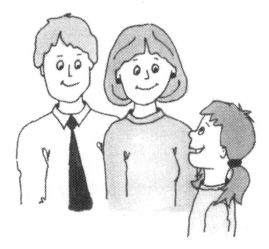

2. Tell your parents about any changes you have with your school schedule. You should also tell them if you are having low blood sugar in school or aren't feeling well.

3. Report to your teacher any insulin or blood sugar changes that might affect you in school. For example, if you have a cold and high blood sugar, you may need more trips to the water fountain and bathroom.

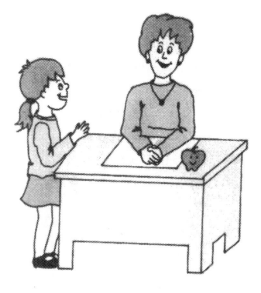

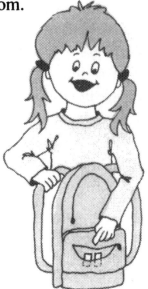

4. Always make sure you have something sweet with you. Don't wait for someone to remind you.

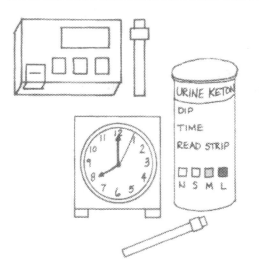

5. Try to do your blood and urine testing without having to be reminded. Moms and Dads really don't like to nag anymore than children like to be nagged. **If you do it first, everyone is happy.** Then, remember to write down your blood sugar and ketone tests.

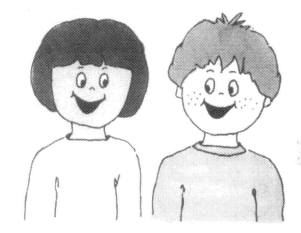

6. Teach other people about your diabetes—especially about low blood sugars. Then they can help if you need them to.

7. It can be fun to go to diabetes camp in the summer. It's a good place to start to learn to be "on your own" and to be with friends.

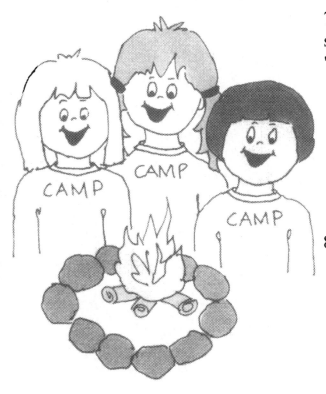

8. Remember your ID bracelet or chain!

Pretty soon you will be an expert in taking care of yourself!

Find these items in the hidden picture.

Syringe   Identification tag   Meter   Testing strip

Cells   Insulin bottle   Pancreas

Name _____ Date _____

Chapter 16.

Friends and Feelings

Sometimes it is hard to have diabetes.

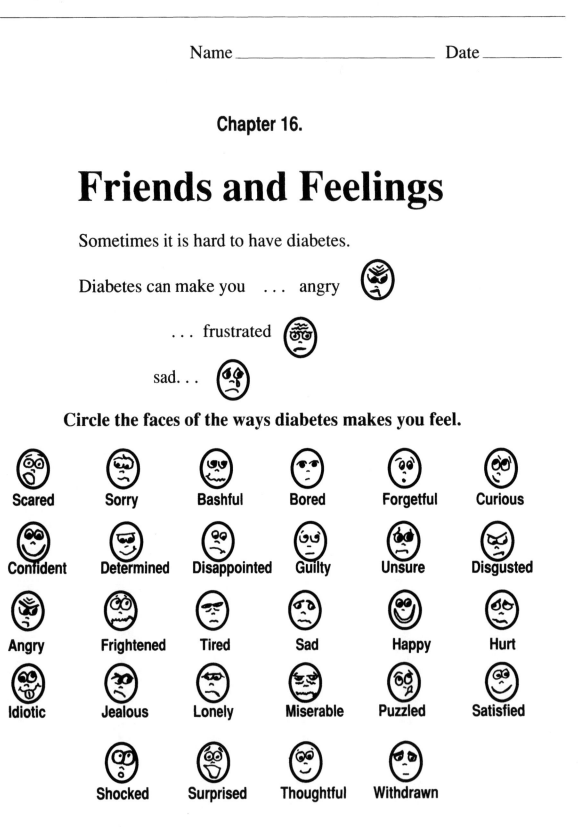

Diabetes can make you . . . angry

. . . frustrated

sad. . .

Circle the faces of the ways diabetes makes you feel.

Scared Sorry Bashful Bored Forgetful Curious

Confident Determined Disappointed Guilty Unsure Disgusted

Angry Frightened Tired Sad Happy Hurt

Idiotic Jealous Lonely Miserable Puzzled Satisfied

Shocked Surprised Thoughtful Withdrawn

How does diabetes make you feel?

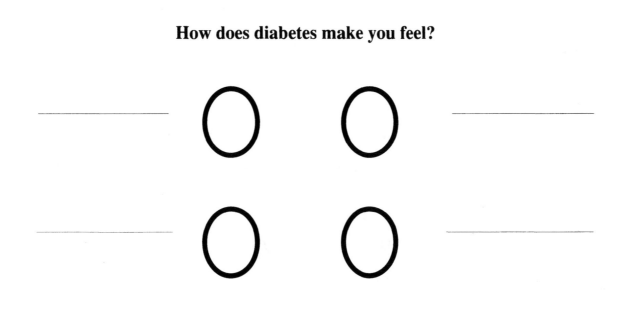

When you have diabetes, sometimes you may wish you wouldn't have to take insulin or do finger sticks. Sometimes you might want to eat or drink foods not on your meal plan, and other times you might not feel like eating things you know you should eat.

You may feel angry or sad. The important thing is to not let your feelings get in the way of taking good care of yourself. The best thing to do is to talk about it with your parents, a good friend, a teacher, or someone who cares. It is OK to feel angry or sad. Everyone who has diabetes feels like you do sometimes.

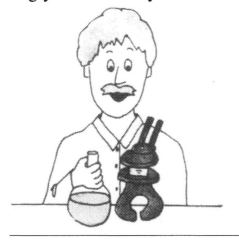

Scientists are trying very hard to find a cure for diabetes. But in the meantime, staying in shape and taking care of yourself will help you do all the things you want to do in your life. And if you learned a lot from this workbook, then you're on the way!

Approximate Blood Sugar Levels in Millimols per Liter (mmol/L)

Certificate of Accomplishment

✳ ✳ ✳ ✳ ✳

This is to certify that

_____

has completed the workbook

It's Time to Learn About Diabetes

_____
(Date)

Signed _____
(Educator)

**You've done a great job!
We're proud of you
for learning about how
to take care of yourself!**

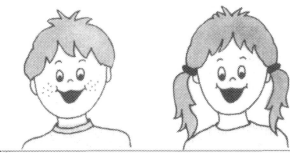

Answers to Workbook Questions

Unit I.

Chapter 1.

Page 14. 1. brain, 2. stomach, 3. pancreas, 4. lungs, 5. heart

Page 16. diabetes

Page 17. 1. pancreas, 2. no, 3. a cold or flu

Page 22. Take insulin, test blood, eat on time, write down your blood and urine sugar numbers, test urine

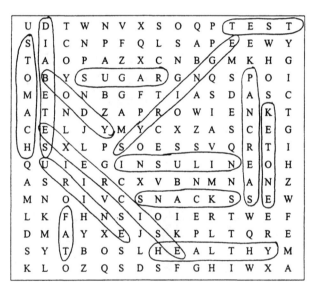

Unit II.

Chapter 2.

Page 26. Pancreas, cells, insulin, sugar

Page 29. Lose weight, go to the bathroom a lot, thirsty, tired

Chapter 3.

Page 32. 1. Fat, 2. Sick, 3. Strip, 4. Before, high, sick, 5. Parents, 6. Sugar-free soda

Unit III.

Chapter 4.

Page 35. 1. Sugar, 2. Cells, 3. Insulin

Page 38. 1. Tell an adult; Check your blood for sugar and your urine for ketones. 2. Blood sugar might be high. 3. b, 4. True, 5. True 6. True

Chapter 5.

Page 45.   Foods crossed out: diet soda, water, celery, sugar-free gelatin.
Connect to High: thirsty, urinating a lot
Connect to Low: shaky, sweaty, nightmares, confused, grouchy

Page 48.   Eat something anyway.
Foods with sugar in them.

Unit IV

Chapter 6.

Page 51.   Regular: begins in 1/2 hour, works fast, clear
NPH or Lente: works slowly, cloudy, works hardest in 8 hours

Page 52.   Squirt it out and start all over again.

Page 55.

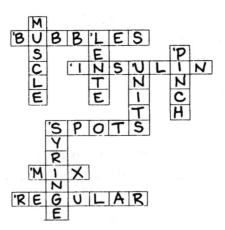

Chapter 8.

Page 62.   Bread: crackers, peas, cereal
Fruit: banana, apples
Meat: cheese, eggs, peanut butter
Milk: milk, yogurt
Vegetable: carrots, lettuce
Fat: nuts, salad dressing

Page 66.   More from all food groups,   1 hour

Chapter 9.

Page 70.   Circle: walking, biking, swimming, baseball, kickball, hockey, basketball, running, tennis, soccer

Chapter 10.

Page 72.   Insulin, Exercise, Food

Page 73.   80,   140,   101

Page 79.   Get up on time, test, take insulin, eat breakfast, go back to sleep.

Unit V.

Chapter 11.

Page 82.

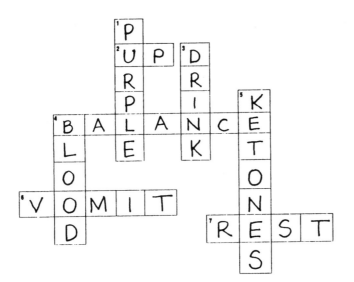

Unit VI.

Chapter 14.

Page 90.

Don't prick—pass disease.

Safely throw out—won't get stuck.

Plastic jug—safely throw in garbage.

Bibliography

Bibace R, Walsh M: New Dimensions for Child Development: Children's Conceptions of Health, Illness, and Bodily Functions. No. 14. San Francisco, Jossey-Bass, December, 1981.

Bigge M: Learning Theories for Teachers, Fourth Edition. Harper & Row Publishers, 1982.

Crider C: Children's Conceptions of the Body Interior. In: Bibace R, Walsh M (Eds): New Directions for Child Development: Children's Conceptions of Health, Illness, and Bodily Functions. No. 14. San Francisco, Jossey-Bass, December, 1981, pages 49-65.

Drash A: Clinical Care of the Diabetic Child. Year Book Medical Publishers, Chicago, 1987.

Fries M: Review of the Literature on the Latency Period. Readings in Psychoanalytic Psychology, Levit M (Ed): Appleton-Century Crofts, New York, 1959, pages 56-69.

Handle With Care: How to Throw Out Used Syringes and Lancets at Home. Environment Law Institute, United States Environmental Protection Agency, Office of Solid Waste, Washington, DC, 1990.

Harrigan J, Faro B, VanPutte A, Stoler P: The Application of Locus of Control to Diabetes Education in School-Aged Children. J Pediat Nursing 24:236-243, 1987.

Puczynski S, Betschart J: Foundation for the Future: Understanding the Student with Diabetes. Greater Pittsburgh Juvenile Diabetes Foundation, American Association of Diabetes Educators, 1991.

Siminerio L, Betschart J: Children with Diabetes. American Diabetes Association, 1986.

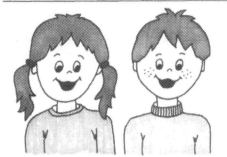

Hi Again! In this workbook, you learned about taking insulin, and how it helps your body use food to give you energy! We use **Humulin®**, an insulin made by the **Lilly Company**.

There are many kinds of insulin! It's really important to never change the kind of insulin you take unless your doctor tells you to.

The **Lilly Company** helps people take care of themselves by giving information to doctors, nurses, and people with diabetes.

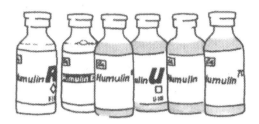

Another company that helps people with diabetes is called **Boehringer Mannheim**. They make meters called **Accu-Chek®** that make it easy to test blood sugar. It

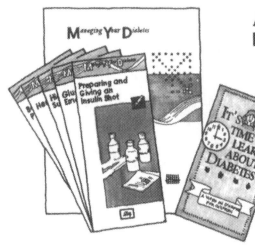

helps us decide how to balance our insulin, food, and exercise. They make different kinds of meters so you can pick one that's just right for

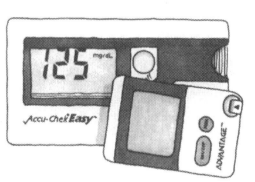

you! **Boehringer Mannheim** has been making strips and meters to test blood sugar for over 20 years.

If you have questions about your diabetes or about **Humulin®** insulin, call your doctor, nurse, drug store, or diabetes care team. Or call **Lilly** at **1-800-545-5979**.

If you have questions about your **Accu-Chek®** meter, you can call **Boehringer Mannheim** 24 hours a day; every day of the year! The number is **1-800-858-8072**.

Take Care of Yourself!

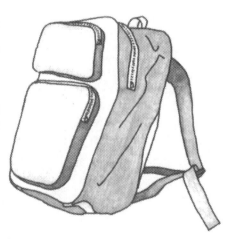

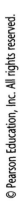

Nombre _____

Fecha _____

Manos a la obra 2 (páginas 360–363)

1 Lee las siguientes palabras y escribe una definición para cada una. Usa el diccionario sólo si es necesario.

1. establecer _Las respuestas variarán_ _____

2. enfrentarse _____

3. luchar _____

4. la tierra _____

5. rebelarse _____

6. desconocido _____

7. adoptar _____

8. los antepasados _____

2 Luego escribe en una hoja aparte, un párrafo en el que uses las palabras anteriores. Recuerda que antes de empezar a escribir tu párrafo, debes pensar en un tema sobre el cual puedas escribir combinando estas palabras. Las respuestas variarán.

Observa las escenas sobre Cortés en las páginas 360 y 361 de tu libro de texto. Contesta las siguientes preguntas. Respuestas posibles.

1. ¿Cómo sabes quién es Cortés en cada pintura?

Lo sé porque lleva una indumentaria diferente a la de los aztecas. _____

2. ¿Cómo crees que se ilustra la relación entre Cortés y los aztecas?

Los aztecas admiran a los conquistadores. _____

3. ¿Qué distingue a los conquistadores en ambas pinturas, aparte del vestuario?

Todos llevan lanzas u otras armas. _____

4. ¿Qué símbolo tienen en común ambas pinturas? ¿En qué se distingue cada una?

Hay un collar de regalo en las dos pinturas. En la de la página 360, los aztecas le

dan el collar a Cortés. En la de la página 361, Cortés le da el collar a uno de los

enviados de Moctezuma. _____

Nombre _____

Fecha _____

El gobierno de los Estados Unidos está formado por diferentes poderes. Cada uno de los poderes del gobierno tiene una función diferente. Completa la siguiente red de palabras con los datos que recuerdes sobre la organización del gobierno de los Estados Unidos y sus funciones.

(página **361**)

Conexiones Las ciencias sociales

GOBIERNO DE
LOS ESTADOS UNIDOS

PODER: _____
REPRESENTANTE: _____
FUNCIONES: _____

PODER: _____
REPRESENTANTE: _____
FUNCIONES: _____

PODER: _____
REPRESENTANTE: _____
FUNCIONES: _____

Las respuestas variarán, pero deberán incluir información sobre los poderes ejecutivo, legislativo y judicial.

En voz alta

Lee el poema *Calabó y bambú* de la sección *En voz alta* prestando especial atención a las palabras que usa el autor. Subraya las palabras que no conozcas así como las palabras que describan sonidos. En una hoja aparte, escribe lo que crees que significa cada palabra. En el caso de las palabras que representan sonidos, identifica a qué cosa o animal pertenece ese sonido. Usa estas palabras para hacer oraciones. Las respuestas variarán.

(página **363**)

Nombre _____ Fecha _____

El español en el mundo del trabajo (página 365)

Los profesionales bilingües son muy útiles en los museos y otras instituciones educativas. Pero hay otros lugares o empleos que necesitan personas que hablen dos o más idiomas. Piensa en cuatro profesiones en las que es muy útil saber más de un idioma. Para cada profesión, indica por qué es importante. Escribe tus respuestas en una hoja aparte.

Las respuestas variarán.

Lee el texto "Mi herencia africana" de la página 362 de tu libro de texto. En una hoja aparte, haz una lista de los distintos elementos que usa la autora para describir su herencia.

Modelo
padre: herencia africana
madre: antepasados españoles e indígenas

Ahora, escribe tu propia versión sobre las culturas de las que está formada tu herencia. Ten en cuenta los elementos que usó la autora en "Mi herencia africana" para hacer tu narración. Cuando termines tu versión, compártela con la clase.

Las respuestas variarán.

Nombre _____ Fecha _____

Fondo cultural (página 362)

En tu libro de texto leíste sobre la comida texmex, que combina la cocina mexicana y la texana. Hoy en día muchos cocineros profesionales mezclan ingredientes de las cocinas de distintas culturas. Inventa tu propio menú de comidas combinadas. Puedes usar los sabores e ingredientes de un país que conozcas y los de cualquier otro país que te interese. Por ejemplo, podrías combinar la hamburguesa estadounidense con la arepa venezolana para formar la "hamburrarepa." Completa el menú de tu nuevo restaurante. Recuerda escribir el nombre del plato así como una breve descripción del mismo.

Restaurante *Las respuestas variarán.*

Aperitivos

Acompañamientos

Platos principales

Postres

Bebidas

Gramática

El imperfecto del subjuntivo

(páginas 364–366)

Como aprendiste anteriormente, usas el subjuntivo para persuadir a otra persona a hacer algo, para expresar emociones acerca de una situación y para expresar duda o incertidumbre. Si el verbo principal está en el tiempo presente, usa el presente del subjuntivo. Si el verbo principal está en el pretérito o el imperfecto, usa el imperfecto del subjuntivo.

Los indígenas **dudan** que los europeos **aprendan** su lengua.
Los indígenas **dudaban** que los europeos **aprendieran** su lengua.

El profesor **sugiere** que **aprendamos** los nombres de las colonias.
El profesor **sugirió** que **aprendiéramos** los nombres de las colonias.

- Para formar el imperfecto del subjuntivo, toma la forma para *Uds./ellos/ellas* en el pretérito y reemplaza la terminación *-ron* por las terminaciones del imperfecto del subjuntivo. A continuación se muestran las formas en el imperfecto del subjuntivo para *cantar, aprender y vivir.*

cantar		aprender		vivir	
cantara	cantáramos	aprendiera	aprendiéramos	viviera	viviéramos
cantaras	cantarais	aprendieras	aprendierais	vivieras	vivierais
cantara	cantaran	aprendiera	aprendieran	viviera	vivieran

- Observa que la forma para *nosotros* lleva acento ortográfico.

Los verbos irregulares, los verbos que cambian la raíz y los verbos con cambios ortográficos siguen la misma regla para formar el imperfecto del subjuntivo.

ir: fueron	→	fue-
haber: hubieron	→	hubie-
pedir: pidieron	→	pidie-
construir: construyeron	→	construye-

El rey les dijo que **fueran** al Nuevo Mundo.
Yo dudaba que **hubiera** semejanzas.
No era necesario que **pidieran** tantas armas.
Los europeos querían que los habitantes **construyeran** una iglesia.

Gramática interactiva

Inténtalo
Lee los últimos cuatro ejemplos de oraciones del recuadro que usan el presente del subjuntivo. Vuelve a escribir cada uno en el presente. Recuerda que en el presente se usa el presente del subjuntivo.

El rey les dice que vayan al Nuevo Mundo.

_____

Dudo que haya semejanzas.

_____

No es necesario que pidan tantas armas.

_____

Los europeos quieren que los habitantes construyan una iglesia.

_____

Recuerda cómo fue la llegada de los españoles y otros exploradores europeos a las Américas a finales del siglo XV. Encierra en un círculo la forma del verbo que corresponda.

1. Los europeos no creían que el imperio azteca **fue** / **fuera** tan poderoso.

2. Los españoles querían que los indígenas **adoptaran** / adoptaron) su religión, su lengua y su cultura.

3. Los reyes católicos querían que los españoles (funden / **fundaran**) una colonia.

4. Nadie pensaba que (**hubiera** / haya) tantas riquezas.

5. No era posible que la cultura de los indígenas (**fuera** / sea) semejante a la de los europeos.

6. Los soldados deseaban que los indígenas les (obedezcan / **obedecieran**).

Imagínate que el año pasado te mudaste con tu familia y empezaste en una escuela nueva. Piensa en las dudas que tendrías sobre los siguientes temas y completa las oraciones usando el imperfecto del subjuntivo. Las respuestas variarán.

- las clases
- los amigos
- los deportes
- los profesores

Modelo   *Deseaba que me aceptaran en el equipo de béisbol.*

1. Tenía miedo de que... _____

2. Dudaba que... _____

3. Esperaba que... _____

4. No estaba seguro(a) de que... _____

Go Online
PHSchool.com

Nombre _____ Fecha _____

Gramática

El imperfecto del subjuntivo con si (páginas 367–369)

Usa el imperfecto del subjuntivo después de si cuando una situación es improbable, imposible o no es verdadera.

Si tuviera tiempo, aprendería más sobre las misiones.
Si viviéramos en México, adoptaríamos las costumbres del país.
Ese imperio sería más poderoso si tuviera oro.

• Observa que usas el imperfecto del subjuntivo después de si y el condicional en la cláusula principal.

Después de como si siempre se debe usar el imperfecto del subjuntivo sin importar el tiempo del primer verbo en la oración. Observa que el otro verbo puede estar en el tiempo presente o en el pasado.

El se vestía como si fuera un rey.
Hablan como si supieran la lengua desde niños.

Gramática interactiva
Más ejemplos
En una hoja aparte, escribe otros dos ejemplos usando el imperfecto del subjuntivo con si.
Las respuestas variarán.

Luis y Marta acaban de salir de una clase y comentan sobre lo que aprendieron. Completa el diálogo con el imperfecto del subjuntivo de los verbos entre paréntesis.

Marta: —¿Te gustó la clase sobre las herencias de nuestro país?
Luis: —Sí, me gustó mucho. Si tuvieras tiempo, quizá _____ estudiara (estudiar) más sobre el tema.
Marta: —¿Sabes cuál es tu herencia?
Luis: —Sé que tengo descendencia europea, pero no estoy seguro. Si _____ pudiera (poder) hablar con mi abuela, lo sabría porque ella tiene toda la información de nuestros antepasados.
Marta: —Si yo _____ fuera (ser) tú, le escribiría mañana mismo una carta.
Luis: —Buena idea ... Ella se pondría muy feliz porque sería como si _____ estuviera (estar) aquí conmigo ayudándome con mis cosas.
Marta: —Si tú _____ quisieras (querer) aquí conmigo, yo te podría ayudar con la carta.
Luis: —Gracias. Me encantaría si tú me _____ ayudaras (ayudar).

256 Capítulo 8 • Gramática

© Pearson Education, Inc. All rights reserved.

Nombre _____ Fecha _____

¿Cómo actuarías en las siguientes situaciones? Lee las siguientes situaciones y explica cómo actuarías tú si te encontraras en ellas.

Modelo Escuchas un idioma desconocido.
Si escuchara un idioma desconocido, preguntaría de dónde es.

1. Un antepasado lejano te viene a visitar a tu casa.
Las respuestas variarán.

2. Viajas a un país con una gran población de indígenas.

3. No sabes nada acerca de tu descendencia.

4. Conoces a un misionero español.

5. Ves a un grupo de personas luchando.

6. Encuentras una cartera en la calle.

Imagina que estuviste presente durante la llegada de los españoles y otros exploradores europeos a las Américas. Recuerda las cosas que sucedieron durante esos tiempos y da tu opinión sobre cómo actuarías tú en el lugar de las personas que participaron en la expedición. Escribe en una hoja aparte cinco oraciones sobre tus ideas. Usa el imperfecto del subjuntivo con si en tus oraciones.
Las respuestas variarán.

Modelo *Si yo fuera soldado, no lucharía contra los indígenas.*

Go Online PHSchool.com

Capítulo 8 Realidades para hispanohablantes 257

© Pearson Education, Inc. All rights reserved.

130 Capítulo 8 – Guía del maestro

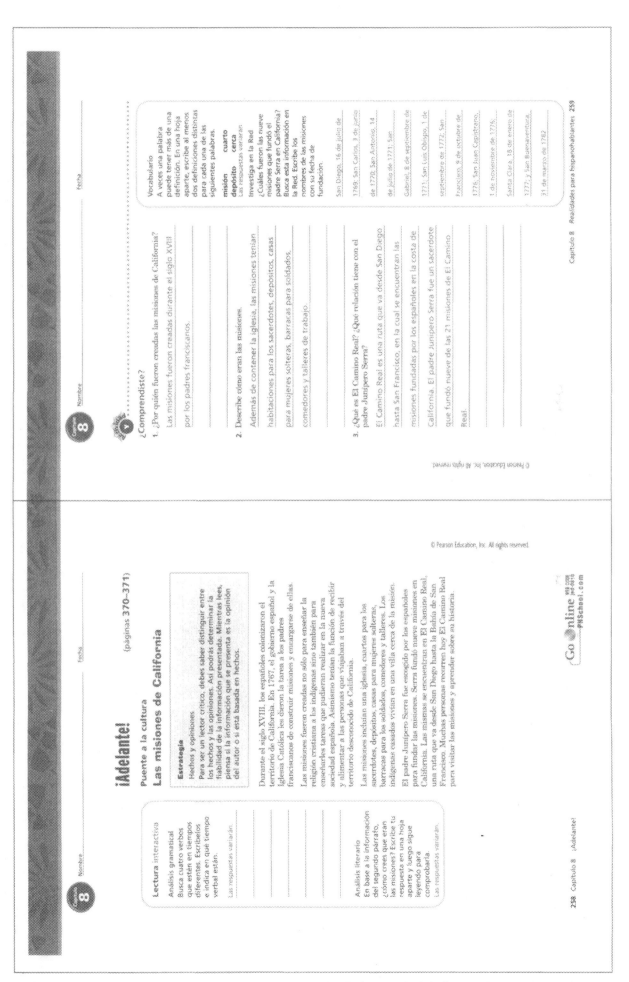

Nombre _____ Fecha _____

¡Adelante! (páginas 370–371)

Puente a la cultura
Las misiones de California

Estrategia

Hechos y opiniones
Para ser un lector crítico, debes saber distinguir entre los hechos y las opiniones. Así podrás determinar la fiabilidad de la información presentada. Mientras lees, piensa si la información que se presenta es la opinión del autor o si está basada en hechos.

Durante el siglo XVIII, los españoles colonizaron el territorio de California. En 1767, el gobierno español y la Iglesia Católica les dieron la tarea a los padres franciscanos de construir misiones y encargarse de ellas.

Las misiones fueron creadas no sólo para enseñar la religión cristiana a los indígenas sino también para enseñarles tareas que pudieran realizar en la nueva sociedad española. Asimismo tenían la función de recibir y alimentar a las personas que viajaban a través del territorio desconocido de California.

Las misiones incluían una iglesia, cuartos para los sacerdotes, depósitos, casas para mujeres solteras, barracas para los soldados, comedores y talleres. Los indígenas casados vivían en una villa cerca de la misión.

El padre Junípero Serra fue escogido por los españoles para fundar las misiones. Serra fundó nueve misiones en California. Las mismas se encuentran en El Camino Real, una ruta que va desde San Diego hasta la Bahía de San Francisco. Muchas personas recorren hoy El Camino Real para visitar las misiones y aprender sobre su historia.

Lectura interactiva

Análisis gramatical
Busca cuatro verbos que estén en tiempos diferentes. Escríbelos e indica en qué tiempos verbal están.
Las respuestas variarán.

Análisis literario
En base a la información del segundo párrafo, ¿cómo crees que eran las misiones? Escribe tu respuesta en una hoja aparte y luego sigue leyendo para comprobarla.
Las respuestas variarán.

Go **O**nline
WEB CODE
jed-0810
PHSchool.com

Nombre _____ Fecha _____

¿Comprendiste?

1. ¿Por quién fueron creadas las misiones de California?

Las misiones fueron creadas durante el siglo XVIII

por los padres franciscanos.

_____

2. Describe cómo eran las misiones.

Además de contener la iglesia, las misiones tenían

habitaciones para los sacerdotes, depósitos, casas

para mujeres solteras, barracas para soldados,

comedores y talleres de trabajo.

_____

3. ¿Qué es El Camino Real? ¿Qué relación tiene con el padre Junípero Serra?

El Camino Real es una ruta que va desde San Diego

hasta San Francisco, en la cual se encuentran las

misiones fundadas por los españoles en la costa de

California. El padre Junípero Serra fue un sacerdote

que fundó nueve de las 21 misiones de El Camino

Real.

_____

Vocabulario
A veces una palabra puede tener más de una definición. En una hoja aparte, escribe al menos dos definiciones distintas para cada una de las siguientes palabras.

misión   cuarto
depósito   cerca
Las respuestas variarán.

Investiga en la Red
¿Cuáles fueron las nueve misiones que fundó el padre Serra en California? Busca esta información en la Red. Escribe los nombres de las misiones con su fecha de fundación.

San Diego, 16 de julio de

1769; San Carlos, 3 de junio

de 1770; San Antonio, 14

de julio de 1771; San

Gabriel, 8 de septiembre de

1771; San Luis Obispo, 1 de

septiembre de 1772; San

Francisco, 9 de octubre de

1776; San Juan Capistrano,

1 de noviembre de 1776;

Santa Clara, 18 de enero de

1777; y San Buenaventura,

31 de marzo de 1782

¿Qué me cuentas? (página 372)

Todos sabemos que las ciudades van cambiando con el pasar de los años. Algunos cambios pueden ser positivos, mientras que otros cambios nos hacen añorar "cómo eran las cosas antes".

Mira las ilustraciones de esta página. Ambas son de la misma ciudad, pero con varias décadas de diferencia. Describe las dos ilustraciones, haciendo énfasis en sus semejanzas y diferencias. Habla sobre detalles históricos y culturales para que tu comparación sea más interesante. Recuerda incluir aspectos positivos y negativos de ambas épocas. Puedes usar los espacios en blanco para escribir notas, pero no puedes usar las notas durante tu presentación. Al hablar ante la clase, haz una pausa luego de explicar cada diferencia y semejanza entre las dos ilustraciones a fin de darles tiempo a tus compañeros de asimilar y entender lo que estás diciendo. Las respuestas variarán.

Estrategia

Comparar y contrastar
Para comparar y contrastar dos elementos, puedes hacer una lista de las cosas que tengan en común y aquellas que sean diferentes. Recuerda que debes concentrarte en varios aspectos de los elementos que vas a comparar, para que la información que presentes sea más interesante.

1.

2.

El Camino Real de California tiene 21 misiones que fueron fundadas para enseñar la religión cristiana a los indígenas. Mira el mapa de El Camino Real que aparece en la página 371 de tu libro de texto. Escoge una de las misiones que aparecen y realiza una investigación sobre la misma. Puedes hacer la investigación en la Red o usar otras fuentes de información. Luego escribe un breve párrafo describiendo su historia y su papel actual y, por último, preséntalo a la clase.

Las respuestas variarán.

8

Presentación oral (página 373)

Imagínate que eres guía turística o en una ciudad multicultural. Vas a guiar a un grupo de turistas que están de visita. Tienes que planear una visita a los lugares más importantes de la ciudad, así como hablar de su historia.

Antes de hacer tu presentación, debes escoger la ciudad en la que organizarás la visita. Puede ser tu ciudad natal, la ciudad donde vives actualmente, una de las ciudades de este capítulo o cualquier otra que te interese. Piensa en las características de la ciudad, su historia, herencia cultural y otros atractivos para los turistas.

Como ayuda, puedes completar una tabla como la que aparece en esta página.

Cuando hagas tu presentación, imagina que tus compañeros de clase son los turistas y que en realidad estás realizando el paseo con ellos. Háblales como lo haría una guía. Usa palabras de uso común y se clara(o) al explicar tus ideas. Probablemente, para tu profesor(a) es importante ver que diste suficiente información sobre la ciudad, que tu presentación fue realista y organizada y que usaste el vocabulario apropiado.

Estrategia

El propósito del presentador
Antes de dar una presentación oral, piensa en la intención de tu discurso. ¿Deseas informar, persuadir o entretener al público? En este caso, tu propósito será el de informar. Necesitas que tu público (los turistas) aprendan algo al mismo tiempo que disfrutan de la visita. Habla sobre detalles interesantes de la ciudad y preséntalos de una manera divertida.

Nombre de la ciudad	Las respuestas variarán.
Historia	
Herencia cultural	
Lugares y edificios importantes	
Restaurantes típicos	
Otros lugares de interés	

8

Presentación escrita (páginas 374–375)

¿Cómo sería ir a vivir a otro país? ¿Alguna vez en tu vida te has mudado de país? ¿Conservan en tu familia las tradiciones de sus antepasados? ¿Conoces a alguien que haya tenido que irse a vivir a otro lugar? Escribe un episodio sobre alguno de estos temas. Puedes escribir sobre tu propia experiencia, la experiencia de alguien que conozcas o puedes inventar una historia.

Antes de empezar a escribir, piensa en lo que deseas contar en la historia. Primero completa la tabla que aparece en esta página para organizar tus ideas. Luego escribe tu borrador en una hoja aparte. Recuerda que debes narrar los eventos en el orden en el que ocurrieron para que tu historia tenga sentido. Añade todos los detalles que sean necesarios y, por último, escribe una versión final en limpio. Las respuestas variarán.

Estrategia

Orden cronológico
Ordenar eventos en orden cronológico significa colocarlos en el orden en que sucedieron. Generalmente esto quiere decir que debes empezar con el primer evento y continuar hasta llegar al último. Pero también puedes usar el orden cronológico invertido, si se adjetiva más a lo que estás relatando. Recuerda usar las expresiones que son indicativas de orden cronológico, como primero, luego, después, segundo, finalmente y por último.

Personaje(s)	Lo que sucedió	Época	Lugar	Pensamientos y sentimientos

Repaso del capítulo

Vocabulario y gramática

para hablar de construcciones
el acueducto — aqueduct
el arco — arch
la arquitectura — architecture
el azulejo — tile
el balcón — balcony
   pl. los balcones
la construcción — construction
la reja — railing, grille
la torre — tower

para hablar de la llegada a las Américas
anteriormente — before
la batalla — battle
el arma pl. las armas — weapon
la colonia — colony
la conquista — conquest
el imperio — empire
el / la indígena — native
la maravilla — marvel, wonder
la misión — mission
el / la misionero(a) — missionary
la población — population
el poder — power
poderoso, -a — powerful
el reto — challenge
la riqueza — wealth
el / la soldado — soldier
la tierra — land

para hablar del encuentro de culturas
africano, -a — African
el antepasado — ancestor
el / la árabe — Arab
cristiano, -a — Christian
la descendencia — descent, ancestry
desconocido, -a — unknown
el encuentro — meeting
la época — time, era
europeo, -a — European

la guerra — war
el grupo étnico — ethnic group
la herencia — heritage
el idioma — language
la influencia — influence
el intercambio — exchange
el / la judío(a) — Jewish
la lengua — language
la mercancía — merchandise
la mezcla — mix
el musulmán, — Muslim
la musulmana
el / la romano(a) — Roman
la raza — race
el resultado — result, outcome
la semejanza — similarity
la unidad — unity
la variedad — variety

verbos
adoptar — to adopt
asimilar(se) — to assimilate
componerse de — to be formed by
conquistar — to conquer
dejar huellas — to leave marks, traces
dominar — to dominate
enfrentarse — to face, to confront
establecer (zc) — to establish
expulsar — to expel
fundar(se) — to found
gobernar (ie) — to rule, to govern
integrarse — to integrate
invadir — to invade
luchar — to fight
ocupar — to occupy
rebelarse — to rebel, to revolt
reconquistar — to reconquer

otras expresiones y palabras
al llegar — upon arriving
maravilloso, -a — wonderful
único, -a — only

---

el condicional
Usa el condicional para expresar lo que harías o cómo sería una situación.

hablar	
hablaría	hablaríamos
hablarías	hablaríais
hablaría	hablarían

ser	
sería	seríamos
serías	seríais
sería	serían

ir	
iría	iríamos
irías	iríais
iría	irían

Los verbos que son irregulares en el futuro tienen las mismas raíces irregulares en el condicional.

tener	
tendría	tendríamos
tendrías	tendríais
tendría	tendrían

Raíces para el futuro y el condicional de otros verbos irregulares:

decir	dir-	poder	podr-	saber	sabr-
haber	habr-	poner	pondr-	salir	saldr-
hacer	har-	querer	querr-	venir	vendr-

el imperfecto del subjuntivo
Usa el subjuntivo para decir lo que una persona pide, espera, cuenta, insiste o requiere de otra. Si el verbo principal está en pretérito o en imperfecto, usa el imperfecto del subjuntivo.

aprender	
aprendiera	aprendiéramos
aprendieras	aprendierais
aprendiera	aprendieran

cantar	
cantara	cantáramos
cantaras	cantarais
cantara	cantaran

vivir	
viviera	viviéramos
vivieras	vivierais
viviera	vivieran

el imperfecto del subjuntivo con si
Usa el imperfecto del subjuntivo después de si cuando una situación sea poco probable, imposible o no sea verdad. Usa el condicional en la cláusula principal.
Si hablaras más, tendrías muchos amigos.
Si Marcos no fuera tan travieso, lo llevaría de paseo.
Usa siempre el imperfecto del subjuntivo después de como si.
Ella se sentía como si estuviera en un lugar desconocido.

● **Más práctica**
Practice Workbook Organizer 8.13, 8.14

Repaso del capítulo

Como preparación para el examen, comprueba que
- sabes la gramática y el vocabulario nuevos
- puedes hacer las tareas de las páginas 265 y 267 de este cuaderno

Preparación para el examen

1 Vocabulario Escribe la letra de la palabra o expresión que mejor complete cada frase.

1. Un ejemplo de un __b__ fue el pueblo romano, porque tuvo tanto poder que pudo decidir el futuro de otros pueblos.
   a. misionero   c. arte
   b. imperio   d. arma

2. Empezó un intercambio de ___ entre Europa y las Américas.
   a. riquezas   c. mercancías
   b. banderas   d. libertad

3. Cuando un país invade a otro país y se queda allí por muchos años, decimos que lo __b__.
   a. expulsa   c. lucha
   b. ocupa   d. permite

4. Como resultado de la mezcla de españoles, indígenas y africanos hay una gran __c__ de culturas en América.
   a. batalla   c. variedad
   b. reja   d. mercancía

5. La Mezquita de Córdoba es un ejemplo de la arquitectura árabe porque tiene muchos ___, igual que la Alhambra, en Granada.
   a. caballos   c. budistas
   b. retos   d. arcos

6. Los misioneros tenían opiniones diferentes sobre ___ de los españoles en la vida de las indígenas.
   a. la semejanza   c. la arquitectura
   b. el azulejo   d. la influencia

7. España era un imperio __b__ en la época de la conquista de América.
   a. único   c. débil
   b. poderoso   d. africano

8. Cuando los cristianos reconquistaron Sevilla, muchos árabes se habían ___ con las españolas.
   a. rebelado   c. asimilado
   b. reconquistado   d. expulsado

2 Gramática Escribe la letra de la palabra o expresión que mejor complete cada frase.

1. Yo __c__ con Luisa por teléfono todos los días si tuviera tiempo, pero estoy muy ocupada.
   a. hablo   c. hablaría
   b. he hablado   d. hablaba

2. Nosotros __b__ al balcón, pero hace mucho frío y está lloviendo.
   a. saldremos   c. saltamos
   b. saldríamos   d. saldrían

3. El arquitecto le dijo al dueño de la casa que ___ el azulejo de color amarillo porque era mejor.
   a. compre   c. comprara
   b. compró   d. compras

4. El rey de España lo miró como si ___ que estaba mintiendo.
   a. creyera   c. creía
   b. crea   d. creerá

5. La madre le dijo al niño que __a__ a la escuela después de comprar la comida.
   a. vendría   c. vinieron
   b. vamos   d. viene

6. "Si __b__ todas tus riquezas, te regalaría mis caballos", le dijo el español al indígena.
   a. me das   c. me diste
   b. me dieras   d. me dieron

7. Aprenderíamos otros idiomas, como el chino, si __a__ la oportunidad de estudiarlos en la escuela.
   a. tuviéramos   c. tuvieran
   b. tuvimos   d. tuvieras

8. Los misioneros querían que los indígenas __d__ su religión.
   a. adoptáramos   c. adoptaran
   b. adoptaran   d. adoptaran

Go Online
PHSchool.com
WEB CODE jed-0811

Consulte las respuestas en la edición del maestro.

En el examen vas a...	Éstas son las tareas de práctica que te pueden ser útiles para el examen...	Si necesitas repasar...
3 Escuchar Escuchar y comprender la descripción de una visita a un pueblo indígena	La visitante describe su visita a un pueblo. (a) ¿Por qué es famoso ese pueblo? ¿Qué dice de la arquitectura? (b) ¿Qué le impresiona más? ¿Qué le recuerda el mercado? (c) ¿Qué otras cosas encuentra allí? (d) ¿Con qué compara al pueblo?	pp. 344–347 *A primera vista 1* p. 347 Actividad 1 p. 350 Actividad 4 p. 354 Actividad 15 p. 379 *Interacción con la lectura*
4 Hablar Presentar una visita guiada para conocer una ciudad	Escoge una ciudad que te guste. Imagina que le hablas de esta ciudad a un recién llegado. Menciona (a) los edificios históricos, (b) las culturas y religiones, (c) una breve historia de la ciudad y (d) lugares donde los jóvenes se divierten.	p. 350 Actividad 8 p. 354 Actividad 15 p. 373 *Presentación oral*
5 Leer Leer y comprender un cuento	Lee este párrafo sobre las aventuras de un indígena azteca y di: (a) ¿En qué ciudad crees que se despierta Maco? ¿En qué época sería? (b) ¿Qué lengua habla la gente? (c) ¿Crees que es un sueño o es la realidad? *Un día, Maco, un joven indígena azteca, cerró sus ojos y cuando los abrió se vio en medio de una ciudad muy diferente a la que vivía. La gente era alta con los cabellos claros. Llevaban ropa larga y zapatos. Hablaban una lengua familiar, parecida a la de las personas que habían llegado a su tierra hacía poco tiempo. La gente lo miraba, pero nadie se paraba a hablarle...*	pp. 376–379 *Lectura*
6 Escribir Escribir una reseña sobre la herencia	Escribe una reseña sobre qué cosas pueden hacer las familias para mantener su herencia cultural y las tradiciones de sus antepasados. Sugiere qué pueden hacer para mantener el idioma, las comidas y otras tradiciones familiares.	p. 351 Actividad 9 p. 351 Actividad 10 pp. 374–375 *Presentación escrita*
7 Pensar Pensar en ejemplos de intercambio cultural en el mundo de hoy y decir si son positivos o no	Da un ejemplo de un intercambio entre culturas en el mundo de hoy en día. Di por qué crees que ese intercambio es positivo o crea conflictos. ¿Crees que ayuda a que las personas se integren o no?	p. 350 Actividad 8 p. 362 Actividad 24 pp. 370–371 *Puente a la cultura*

Nombre _____ Fecha _____

Capítulo 9

Cuidemos nuestro planeta (páginas 388–389)

Objetivos del capítulo

- Hablar sobre cuestiones medioambientales en la comunidad
- Hablar sobre cómo resolver problemas del medio ambiente a nivel local y global
- Expresar actitudes y opiniones sobre el medio ambiente
- Comprender diferentes perspectivas culturales acerca de la conservación y el medio ambiente

Fondo cultural

1 Mira el mural *Creación* de Diego Rivera e identifica dos elementos que ves en el cuadro. Después mira el detalle del otro mural de Rivera, el del Detroit Institute of Arts, sobre el que leíste en la página 219 de tu libro de texto. ¿Qué elementos ves en el cuadro?

Creación	Detroit Institute of Arts
Las respuestas variarán.	

2 Para ti, ¿son opuestos los temas de los dos murales? ¿Por qué? ¿Crees que sea posible encontrar un equilibrio entre el mundo natural y el mundo industrial? Escribe tus ideas abajo. Las respuestas variarán.

_____
_____
_____
_____

¿Sabes qué problemas ambientales tienen en el país de tu herencia cultural? Investiga o pregunta a tus familiares sobre lo que ocurre allí con el medio ambiente. En una hoja aparte, haz una lista de los problemas principales y lo que hace la gente para resolverlos. Las respuestas variarán.

Go Online WEB CODE jed-0902 PHSchool.com

Capítulo 9 Realidades para hispanohablantes 269

Nombre _____ Fecha _____

Capítulo 9

A ver si recuerdas . . . (páginas 384–387)

El medio ambiente es un tema sobre el que muchas personas tienen opiniones firmes. ¿Qué piensas tú sobre asuntos como el reciclaje, los efectos del tráfico, los recursos naturales y los animales en peligro de extinción? Expresa tus opiniones a continuación empezando con las frases indicadas. Consulta el vocabulario en las páginas 384 y 386 de tu libro de texto como ayuda.

El medio ambiente

Me importa(n) . . . .

Las respuestas variarán.

_____
_____

Me interesa(n) . . . .

_____
_____

Me molesta(n) . . . .

_____
_____

Me parece(n) . . . .

_____
_____

Me preocupa(n) . . . .

_____
_____

Me encanta(n) . . . .

_____
_____

Me gusta(n) . . . .

_____
_____

Go Online WEB CODE jed-0901 PHSchool.com

268 Capítulo 9 A ver si recuerdas . . .

Nombre _____ Fecha _____

A primera vista 1 (páginas 390-393)

Haz una lista para cada uno de los siguientes aspectos. Las respuestas variarán.

1. Cosas que podrían suceder tan pronto como se agoten los recursos de energía:

_____
_____

2. Recursos naturales que podemos usar:

_____
_____

3. Cosas de las que hay escasez:

_____
_____

4. Cosas de las que dependemos:

_____
_____

Busca sinónimos o expresiones equivalentes para las palabras o frases siguientes.
Después escribe una oración usando cada una de las expresiones originales.

1. tan pronto como   en cuanto, enseguida que
   Las respuestas variarán. _____

2. estar a cargo de   encargarse de, estar al mando de
   Las respuestas variarán. _____

3. agotarse   terminarse, acabarse
   Las respuestas variarán. _____

4. desperdiciar malgastar, usar más de lo debido
   Las respuestas variarán. _____

Nombre _____ Fecha _____

Ampliación del lenguaje

Las siglas

En el texto de la página 393 de tu libro de texto has aprendido qué es el ICPRO. Estas siglas pertenecen a la organización Industria y Comercio Pro-Reciclaje, de Puerto Rico. Mucha gente usa las siglas de una organización para no tener que pronunciar nombres demasiado largos. Las siglas, generalmente, toman la primera letra de cada una de las palabras del nombre. Por lo tanto, los acrónimos varían del español al inglés. Puedes estar familiarizado con un acrónimo en inglés, y no saber su equivalente en español, y viceversa. Algunos acrónimos de uso común son la ONU (Organización de las Naciones Unidas, que en inglés es la UN), la OEA (Organización de Estados Americanos, OAS, en inglés), o la UE (Unión Europea, EU, en inglés).

Escoge una de las organizaciones que se mencionan arriba y describe cuál es su labor. Puedes trabajar con un(a) compañero(a) de clase para generar ideas. Después, compartan sus ideas con el resto de la clase.

Las respuestas variarán. _____

_____
_____
_____
_____
_____
_____
_____
_____

Go Online
PHSchool.com

Nombre _____ Fecha _____

Manos a la obra 1 (páginas 394–397)

Ampliación del lenguaje

Diptongos e hiatos

Se forman **diptongos** cuando una vocal fuerte (a, e, o) se une con una vocal débil (i, u) no acentuada. También forman diptongo la combinación de dos vocales débiles distintas. En un diptongo, se pronuncian las dos vocales en una sola sílaba.

recipiente   desperdicio   agua   suficiente   gobierno

Una h intercalada entre dos vocales que formen diptongo no impide que se forme el diptongo.

ahumar   ahijado

Forman **hiatos** dos vocales juntas que se pronuncian en sílabas separadas. Estas vocales pueden ser una combinación de dos vocales fuertes (caer, océano) o una vocal fuerte y una débil tónica: (día, reúne)

Lee las siguientes oraciones. Pon un círculo alrededor de los diptongos y subraya los hiatos que encuentres.

1. Es peor para el ambiente usar productos que causan contaminación.

2. He oído que el gobierno no quiere tomar medidas para reducir el ruido en la ciudad.

3. No deberíamos echar basura ni desperdicios al océano.

4. La población no sabe si habrá suficientes recursos naturales en el futuro.

5. Recibí un correo sobre la protección del medio ambiente.

6. Las científicas estudian las posibles repercusiones del aumento de la temperatura promedio en la Tierra.

272 Capítulo 9 · Manos a la obra 1

Nombre _____ Fecha _____

Contesta las siguientes preguntas sobre los problemas del medio ambiente.

1. ¿Cuál crees que es el principal problema del medio ambiente en tu comunidad?
Las respuestas variarán.

2. ¿Qué medidas piensas que se deberían tomar para solucionarlo?

3. ¿Estarías a favor o en contra de la restricción de vehículos en tu área? ¿Por qué?

4. ¿Cuál crees que será el primer recurso que se agotará en el futuro? ¿Por qué?

5. ¿Qué haces tú para ayudar a proteger el medio ambiente?

También se dice . . .

Escribe otras palabras y expresiones que conozcas para hablar sobre los problemas y las soluciones para la protección del medio ambiente.

Las respuestas variarán.

Capítulo 9 · Realidades para hispanohablantes 273

© Pearson Education, Inc. All rights reserved.

138 Capítulo 9 – Guía del maestro

Fondo cultural

(página 396)

En la página 396 de tu libro de texto leíste sobre la "restricción vehicular" en la ciudad de Santiago de Chile. En otras partes del mundo, muchas ciudades están tratando de combatir el problema de la contaminación del aire causada por el excesivo número de coches. Lee a continuación algunos de los planes preparados para reducir el número de coches por las calles de una ciudad imaginaria. ¿Cuáles crees que son las ventajas y desventajas de cada uno de los planes? Las respuestas variarán.

Ventajas	Descripción del plan	Desventajas
	días de uso según el último número de la patente	
	cobrar por usar las calles más transitadas	
	prohibir los coches en el centro de la ciudad	
	mejorar el sistema de transporte público	

¿Cuál de los planes de arriba tiene más sentido en tu opinión? ¿Por qué?

Las respuestas variarán.

_____

_____

_____

_____

_____

Gramática

(páginas 398–401)

Conjunciones que se usan con el subjuntivo y el indicativo

Ciertas conjugaciones relacionadas con el tiempo van seguidas por un verbo en modo indicativo o subjuntivo.

después (de) que	cuando
en cuanto	mientras
	tan pronto como	hasta que

Usamos el modo subjuntivo después de estas conjunciones si la acción que sigue aún no ha ocurrido.

Van a seguir contaminando **hasta que** el gobierno los **castigue**.

Habrá menos contaminación **cuando haya** menos fábricas.

Usamos el indicativo después de estas conjunciones si la acción que sigue ya ha ocurrido u ocurre regularmente.

Siempre apagamos las luces **en cuanto salimos** del cuarto.

• La conjunción **antes de que** va siempre seguida por el subjuntivo.
La empresa cerró **tan pronto como** se pasó grave el problema.

Siempre se agitan los boletos **antes de que yo compre** el mío.

• Si el sujeto de la oración es el mismo, usamos el infinitivo después de **antes de**, **después de** y **hasta**.

Después de visitar (nosotros) la fábrica, debemos escribir el informe. Marisa no piensa descansar **hasta resolver** (ella) el problema.

Gramática interactiva

Más ejemplos

En una hoja aparte, escribe cuatro oraciones con las conjunciones del recuadro. Usa el indicativo en dos de ellas y el subjuntivo en las otras dos.

En una hoja aparte, escribe dos oraciones con conjunciones en las que el sujeto no cambie. Indica cuál es el sujeto de cada oración. Las respuestas variarán.

Ya has leído sobre algunos problemas que afectan al medio ambiente. Demuestra tus conocimientos sobre el tema completando las frases de una conferencia del Dr. Fuente.

modelo *Las aguas estarán contaminadas hasta que dejemos de echar desperdicios.*

1. Las fábricas van a seguir arrojando pesticidas a los ríos hasta que Las respuestas variarán.

_____

2. Tendremos que buscar otras fuentes de energía cuando _____

_____

3. Debemos acabar con la contaminación tan pronto como _____

_____

4. Los peces del río comenzarán a morir en cuanto _____

_____

Estrategia

Escribir a partir de un bosquejo

Cuando usas un bosquejo para escribir, recuerda que cada punto importante del bosquejo te indica el comienzo de un párrafo nuevo. La oración principal del párrafo debe hacer referencia al tema del punto principal y los puntos subordinados deben usarse para desarrollar el párrafo.

(página 401)

1. Imagina que estás haciendo una investigación sobre la lluvia ácida para escribir un artículo en el periódico de tu escuela. Usa el bosquejo de abajo para escribir tu artículo en una hoja aparte. También puedes buscar más información en la biblioteca o en la Red.

Conexiones Las ciencias

I. Causas y efectos de la lluvia ácida
  A. Causada por dióxido de azufre y óxido de nitrógeno
    1. Resultante de plantas generadoras
    2. Aumenta por el efecto del sol
  B. Afecta a los recursos naturales
    1. Ríos, lagos, océanos
      a. peces
      b. otros animales
    2. Bosques
  C. Afecta a los seres humanos
    1. Enfermedades respiratorias
    2. Otras consecuencias
II. Recomendaciones para reducir la lluvia ácida
  A. En el hogar
    1. Disminuir el consumo eléctrico
    2. Evitar el uso de aires acondicionados
  B. Fuera del hogar
    1. Reducir el uso de automóviles
    2. Comprar productos más ecológicos

Modelo

La lluvia ácida es un problema ambiental que nos afecta a todos. Está causada por...
Las respuestas variarán.

---

1. En la sección *Ampliación del lenguaje* de la página 399 de tu libro de texto viste algunos ejemplos de familias de palabras. Lee las palabras de la tabla que aparece a continuación y completa las familias de palabras. Respuestas posibles.

Sustantivos	Adjetivos	Verbos
crecimiento	crecido	crecer
escasez	escaso	escasear
conservación	conservador	conservar
daño	dañado, dañino	dañar
desecho	desechable	desechar
veneno	venenoso	envenenar
agotamiento	agotado	agotar

2. Mira tu lista de vocabulario para este tema y completa las dos últimas líneas de la tabla con dos familias de palabras de tu elección.

3. En una hoja aparte, escribe cinco oraciones sobre el cuidado del medio ambiente usando en cada una de ellas palabras de la tabla y una expresión del siguiente recuadro. Las respuestas variarán.

después de que	mientras	cuando
tan pronto como	hasta que	en cuanto

Modelo

A —*Cuando las aguas de los ríos están envenenadas, no sé qué vamos a hacer.*
B —*Bueno, no podemos esperar hasta que llegue esa situación.*
Conclusión: *Debemos evitar la contaminación de los ríos.*
Las respuestas variarán.

Go Online PHSchool.com WEB CODE jed-0903

Estrategia

Hallar las ideas principales

Cuando escribes algo es necesario que tengas una idea principal que mantenga la unidad de todo el trabajo. Revisa los detalles que has compilado y escribe una oración simple que resuma tu idea o punto principal. Usa esta oración como parte central de un párrafo de introducción. Luego escribe párrafos de apoyo que desarrollen tu punto principal.

Trabaja con otros(as) dos estudiantes. Lee la carta que escribiste en el ejercicio anterior a tus compañeros(as) y coméntala. Luego, escucha con atención las cartas de tus compañeros y escribe un informe sobre qué cosas hacen en general los jóvenes del país. Mientras tus compañeros leen sus cartas, puedes anotar las ideas principales y los detalles importantes que ayuden a describir a los jóvenes.

Las respuestas variarán.

Go Online
PHSchool.com

Gramática

Los pronombres relativos que, quien y lo que (páginas 402–403)

Usamos los pronombres relativos para combinar dos oraciones o para dar información que aclare el significado de la oración. El pronombre relativo más común en español es que y sirve para referirse a personas, animales y cosas.

Ésta es la fábrica **que** visité ayer.
La fábrica, **que** hace productos químicos, fomenta la protección del medio ambiente.
El Sr. Ríos es el profesor **que** nos llevó a la fábrica.

Después de una preposición, usamos que para referirnos a cosas y quien(es) para referirnos a personas.

No encuentro el papel **en que** escribí tu dirección.
El problema **del que** se habló ocurrió en otro barrio.
La señora **a quien** te presenté trabaja en una fábrica de recipientes.

* Usamos la frase relativa lo que para referirnos a una situación, concepto, acción u objeto aún no identificado.

No recuerdo **lo que** me dijo.
Lo que más me gusta es estar a cargo del proyecto.

Gramática interactiva

Inténtalo
En una hoja aparte, escribe una oración con el pronombre relativo que, otra con una preposición y quien(es) y otra con la frase relativa lo que.
Las respuestas variarán.

Tú le quieres escribir una carta a un(a) chico(a) de otro país que viene a pasar un mes en tu casa. Le quieres dar toda la información posible sobre tu familia, tus amigos, lo que haces, tus planes, etc. Escribe seis oraciones usando los pronombres relativos que, quien y lo que.

Modelo: *Lo que más me gustaría hacer cuando vinieras es ir a visitar el parque natural que está cerca de mi ciudad.*

Las respuestas variarán.

9

Nombre _____ Fecha _____

A primera vista 2 (páginas 404–407)

Escribe en tus propias palabras lo que quieren decir las siguientes expresiones.
Después lee tus explicaciones a tus compañeros.

Las respuestas variarán.

1. recalentamiento global _____

2. derrame de petróleo _____

3. en peligro de extinción _____

4. tomar conciencia _____

Completa el siguiente correo electrónico con la palabra o frase adecuada del
vocabulario de esta lección.

Querido Gustavo:

Estoy muy preocupada por los problemas de nuestro planeta. El _____ clima
está cambiando en todo el mundo. El _____ efecto invernadero _____ ha hecho que la
temperatura de muchas regiones aumente y esto está afectando el hábitat de
muchas especies, que ahora están _____ en peligro de extinción _____.
A menos que _____ hagamos algo, la situación no va a mejorar. Por eso he
decidido participar como voluntaria de Greenpeace. Mi primera labor va a ser
colaborar en la _____ limpieza _____ de las playas de Galicia, después del
derrame de petróleo _____ rescatar _____ de hace unos meses. ¿No te gustaría participar a ti
también y ayudar a _____ animales de esa región? Espero que te
animes y vengas a hacer el viaje conmigo.

Besos de tu amiga,

Peggy

9

Nombre _____ Fecha _____

Lee el texto de la página 406 de tu libro de texto. Haz una lista de los términos
científicos que desconoces o que te resulten difíciles. Luego, completa la tabla de abajo
para hacer un glosario científico con las explicaciones de cada uno de estos términos.
Las respuestas variarán.

Término	Explicación

¿Cuál es el parque o reserva natural más cercano a tu comunidad? Haz una
investigación en la Red y averigua la siguiente información:

* nombre del parque o reserva
* lugar donde está
* especies en peligro de extinción
* problemas ecológicos a los que se enfrenta
* programas educativos sobre el parque o reserva

En una hoja aparte, organiza tus averiguaciones en uno o dos párrafos y léelos
a la clase. Si puedes, incluye alguna fotografía o mapa del lugar.
Las respuestas variarán.

Go Online
PHSchool.com